Case Management in
Homeopathic Medicine

*Best practice / Traditional principles and techniques
distilled from 200 years of case management in
Homeopathy for better clinical results*

Alastair C. Gray

Homeopathic Essence

CASE MANAGEMENT IN HOMEOPATHIC MEDICINE

First Edition: 2014
Second Edition: 2018
2nd Impression: 2024

All rights reserved. No part of this book may be reproduced, stored in a retrieval system or transmitted, in any form or by any means, mechanical, photocopying, recording or otherwise, without any prior written permission of the publisher.

© with the author

Published by Kuldeep Jain for
Homeopathic Essence
An Imprint of
Published by Kuldeep Jain for
B. JAIN PUBLISHERS (P) LTD.
D-157, Sector-63, NOIDA-201307, U.P. (INDIA)
Tel.: +91-120-4933333 • Email: info@bjain.com
Website: www.bjainbooks.com
Registered office: 1921/10, Chuna Mandi, Paharganj,
New Delhi-110 055 (India)

Printed in India

ISBN: 978-81-319-3300-8

Foreword

This book, *Case Management in Homeopathic Medicine*, and its companion, *Realities of Contemporary Homeopathy Practice* are excellent sequels to Alastair's first two books *Case Taking* and *Method*.

He covers more of the glorious landscape of homeopathic medicine in leaps and bounds, and in a way that is both fresh and refreshing.

Gray examines case management from a historical perspective combing through the wise counsel of our philosophical giants from Hahnemann, Kent and Close to Vithoulkas, Sherr and Little. He thinks them through using the realities of his own homeopathic practice as a benchmark, to evaluate and re-evaluate each aphorism, each principle.

Gray explores the principles in the context of the often neglected territory of the relationship: between practitioner and patient, between practitioner and practice, between practitioner and profession. Gray questions many of our received wisdoms and often-taught practice management procedures, examining their strengths and weaknesses through numerous case examples including his own. His candidness about his own process and development make this book both accessible and authentic.

Volumes III and IV are designed to be read in tandem. They cover similar territory but in different ways. This volume focusses on traditional case management from a historical perspective. The second volume (IV) brings the topic into the present day by focussing on contemporary case management and complex patient management situations. Think of this book as setting the scene.

I wish I had this book when I was starting out in practice. I would have instituted an annual audit of my practice from the get go. I started doing so when I had been in practice for about five years - out of desperation to know whether I was doing as badly as it seemed I might be. I wasn't. I found out I could hold my head up in public - that I was helping a respectable percentage of the people who were coming to see me. I have conducted clinical audits in my practice on a regular basis since then and found them an invaluable touchstone. I use those times to reflect on my practice as a whole, to identify the parts that are working well, the ones that need some tweaking and those that are more seriously out of sorts and need attention.

Gray discusses his own practice audit experience and how valuable it was for him. He was surprised to find that 93% of his patients were consulting other health care practitioners as well as himself. He uses this information to think about the gap between how homeopathy is taught (as a stand-alone modality) and how patients are increasingly using us (as part of a healing team), between his goals and expectations (for cure) and his patients' (for pain relief).

Gray brings clarity, logic and a deeper understanding to this whole subject. He is surprisingly not dogmatic. He explains a road map for reflecting on case management issues giving coherent ways to think and make decisions. He talks about many difficult aspects of case management. In so doing he encourages flexibility in thinking and practice - encouraging the reader to think homeopathically and rigorously.

Alastair throws down more than a few challenges to the homeopathic profession as a whole. I sincerely hope that this book will generate reflection, and discussion – and above all changes. Changes that reflect the times and many cultures we are living and working within. Changes especially in education to better help this glorious profession evolve.

There's food for thought for all including students, practitioners, educators and researchers. Gray's easy writing style, his unabashed honesty in describing his own challenges, his straightforward sharing of his experiences and inner processes - these all contribute to an unusually enjoyable reading and learning experience.

Miranda Castro
FSHom, RSHom(NA), CCH
Gainesville, Florida 2013

Author, *The Complete Homeopathy Handbook, Homeopathy for Pregnancy, Birth and Your Baby's First Years* (Homeopathy for Mother and Baby), and *A Homeopathic Guide to Stress*
www.mirandacastro.com

Introduction to the Series

- Critical Thinking
- The Need for Clarity
- Scope of Practice
- Homeopathy in Trouble and Under Attack
- The Change in Emphasis within Homeopathic Education
- Research

Introduction to the Series

Critical Thinking

This is the third in a series of books casting a critical eye over the discipline of homeopathic medicine. It is important to note that the critical evaluation is coming from one who is inside the profession. Usually the critiques come from without and often lack an understanding of the historical and other contextual issues. In the scientific and academic world critical analysis, critical reflection and critical evaluation are the solid underpinnings and foundations of any meaningful area of enquiry. It is not necessarily a personal or professional attack.

The Need for Clarity

In this series of books, seven aspects of the practice of homeopathic medicine are examined, reflected on, deconstructed, critically evaluated and described. This last point, 'described' is crucial. Homeopathic medicine from the inside is a stimulating and exciting discipline to be a part of. From the outside it can seem bewildering. Not only because some of the fundamentals of the art and science of homeopathy are difficult to describe in what is clearly and unequivocally a biomedical world. But it is overwhelmingly confusing because of the certain different styles of practice that homeopaths have. This is not just about bedside manner. The user of homeopathy in India may not be so concerned about the method used by the prescriber. The choice of going to this practitioner or that doctor is a simple one. But in the Western world, in Europe, the US, in Australia and New Zealand homeopathy struggles at times because of its breadth and startling difference in the way in which it is carried out.

Scope of Practice

One of the challenges of the profession is that there is no clear scope of practice, clear guidelines on best practice, or exclusivity of title, as at the moment in those countries where homeopathy is unregulated anyone can call themselves a homeopath. This issue of scope practice is a serious problem in the homeopathic world. For a physician, clear directives are given in medical school on how to take a case. In physiotherapy there is a clear path and guidelines. For an auditor going into a business or an educational auditor going into a college there are clear questions to ask and a protocol. Homeopathy has a breadth that makes this very difficult. Because homeopathy is the application of an idea, not merely the distribution of medicines, there is a massive range of application. Homeopathy means, 'similar suffering'. This is the origin of the word that Hahnemann coined. That substance from the natural world that can create symptoms in a healthy person will have the capacity to remove those symptoms in a patient. That is the proposition, yet ask members of the general public what constitutes homeopathic medicine, generally they will identify the issue of the infinitesimal dose, or the fact that homeopaths use serial dilutions of poisons as their therapeutic interventions. Yet the reality is that the infinitesimal dose is secondary to the principle law of homeopathy which is that of the application of similars. This broad scope is the crux of the issue. Homeopathy simply has a massive scope of practice. It is its greatest boon and its largest catastrophe. In a nutshell, there is no symptom of any patient on the planet for which there is not a substance somewhere in nature that has the capacity to create that same symptom in a healthy person. No other profession has such a wide terrain. Homeopaths assert that they can cure everything from depression, heartache, teething pain, lice and herpes. From the perspective of other professions these are bold claims indeed. Furthermore, there is general bewilderment from those looking towards the homeopathic profession that in addition to making these claims there are no agreed guidelines of method or case taking.

It is only possibly the psychological arts and sciences that has anything close to the largeness of scope that homeopaths have. On the one hand you have Psychiatry with its very specific doses of drugs to manage the neuro-chemistry of a patient and it's measurable outcomes, and at the other end of the spectrum you have Somatic Therapy, Gestalt Therapy or Neuro-linguistic Programming. That is a broad scope of strategies and theories orientated to create change in a patient.

In the Western world homeopathy experienced a massive amount of growth in the 1980's and 90's. Private colleges sprang up across Europe, New Zealand, Australia, the US and the unlikeliest of places. Those classrooms were full of the most diverse range of students from interested housewives through to immunologists, physicians, historians, nurses and hippies. Credit where it's due. This was for the most part due to be charismatic and solid work of George Vithoulkas who taught, wrote, published, and raised the awareness of thousands worldwide. A great many were drawn to his lectures and seminars and books. That is a far cry from what we see today at the end of the first decade of the 21st century. Classrooms are still full but they are smaller classrooms. Students are committed but there's no doubt that the student of 2013 is different from the student of 1983.

Homeopathy in Trouble and Under Attack

Modern students hear their teachers talk nostalgically about the old days before the attacks. Skeptics rally outside pharmacies that sell homeopathy, products are recalled, poorly written government reports diminishing good homeopathy research are published. Homeopathy students these days hear their teachers talking about disunity and an implosion from the inside. Comparisons are made to the decline of homeopathy in the US in the early part of the 20th century, 100 years ago where the fledgling profession with students, colleges and hospitals, in the shadow of the Flexner Report, within a generation was almost was swept away and what remained became a cottage industry.

The internal divisions aside, from the outside there are a number of obvious criticisms of homeopathic medicine. Never have they been more sharply defined and focussed than in the UK and Australia over the last five years. Systematic and orchestrated attacks have been launched about non-evidence-

Introduction to the Series   xiii

based medicine (i.e. homeopathy) being free to the public and delivered in the National Health Service (NHS) in the UK, while in Australia the NHMRC report into Homeopathy has bought to bear significant pressure there. Furthermore the profession has withstood criticisms of homeopathy taught in universities, a 'non-science' being taught in science degrees. 'It couldn't possibly work, therefore it doesn't work', has been the cynical message.

All of these recent events have fed perceptions driven by the opponents of homeopathy that it is in the business of taking advantage of vulnerable people, flogging meaningless medicine without conscience, practicing pseudo-science without rigour. How do these perceptions come about? Without doubt ignorance and prejudice on behalf of some, but equally without doubt because of average prescribing, poor practice, negative publicity, because homeopaths have been lazy and have lacked significant academic rigour. With the upsurge in the ability to publish quickly and easily, and with the ability to blog and have an opinion about everything, a great deal of what has emerged in the homeopathic body of literature in the last 20 years has been at the softer end of the spectrum. A word search on 'homeopathy' in Google leads to some bewildering sites and opinions. The number of peer reviewed industry journals are few. This has to change if the profession is to make any progress. These books are an attempt to right the balance, not in a way that is uncritical and reactionary but in a grounded way that seeks to place aspects of homeopathy in their true context.

This volume examines the landscape of homeopathic case management in all of its complexity. To students of homeopathy and those questioning homeopathy this book seeks to describe and identify the varieties that exist within the profession, and just why they are there. Because this discipline spans 200 years and involves a literature base that takes into account the whole globe there is no shortage of variety.

Later volumes will describe the landscape of homeopathic education. These works will focus on the homeopathic community and profession, all at once taking into account the history, the personalities and the evolution of this discipline and ask, 'How Did We Get To This Place?'

My own approach to homeopathy is a fairly grounded one. 'Feet on the ground, head in the clouds' (Sherr 1994), is the best and natural posture to adopt in practice. Homeopathy attracts individualistic people. It attracts creative people, and people that are on their third careers. It attracts people that have been in nursing, or the corporate world and are looking for something else. It also attracts people that are great healers not necessarily great researchers or technicians and certainly not scientists. Homeopathic colleges experience their greatest attrition because of medical sciences subjects not homeopathic ones.

That does not mean my approach to homeopathic medicine is dry by any means. But it does mean one thing in particular and not all homeopaths will be in agreement. After 30 years of practice and 20 years of teaching I'm no longer of the opinion that the homeopathic remedy is the most crucial thing in a positive curative intervention. There has been a heavy emphasis on the remedy as the thing that does the work in the 200 year history of homeopathy. The emphasis has been on the simillimum, the Holy Grail, the silver bullet, the perfect remedy. This detracts from the ultimate skill behind practicing homeopathy. Moreover the idea is divorced from the reality at the coal face of homeopathic practice. It is the therapeutic relationship, and the ability of a homeopath to listen and receive a full case that is at the heart of the good prescription. It is this relationship between the practitioner and the patient that is the true emphasis. When I was in my role as head of the homeopathy department at Endeavour College of Natural Health it was the educational and pedagogical focus. This is not to detract from knowledge of materia medica, theory or philosophy but to right an imbalance.

The Change in Emphasis within Homeopathic Education

A decade ago I was a part of a great team that worked tirelessly to develop the degree curriculum at Endeavour in Australia. While nothing is ever perfect, it was a big step forward. In addition, I worked on the degree submission at Cyberjaya University College of Medical Sciences in Malaysia. Benchmarked against the University of Central Lancashire's undergraduate degree, to my mind these efforts have taken homeopathic medicine education a few necessary steps forward by adding the necessary components of critical thinking iand research. Not all like them or appreciate them. To some these changes are a threat, they represent competition, and they definitely raise the standards to a level that means that some will not be able to attain what is necessary.

Homeopathic education not as aligned as it could be (Gray 2012, 2012b, 2014). In colleges and schools world-wide there is a disconnect about professional standards, in other words, what is agreed upon as the necessary skills to develop in order to competently practice homeopathic medicine, and the level to which these subjects are taught. Diplomas and advanced diplomas get clogged with massive amounts of critical thinking and cognitive skills that are educationally well ahead of the award they are offering. There is over-assessment. Outside the colleges, homeopathic education is driven by entrepreneurs not educators, large personalities with an angle attempt to keep students coming back with the next thing.

We have thousands upon thousands of cured cases, that are passed on from practitioner to teacher, teacher to student, and over the years many of these have found their way into our journals. Uncomfortable and distressing as it is, in the 21st century, in the biomedical world in which we live, these constitute nothing but anecdotal evidence. In the cold world of science, anecdotal evidence sits at the very bottom of the evidence hierarchy. At the top of the evidence hierarchy is the systematic review, and then the gold standard randomised controlled double-blind trial. There are some but precious few of these in homeopathy and just one of these trials counts for more than thousands upon thousands of anecdotal stories. Practicing homeopaths find this an unhappy situation to find themselves in. Some deal with it by saying, 'Well that cold scientific world is stuffed and they can have it. We don't have to play their games and play in that biomedical sandpit. We will do our own thing'. Some decide to become more medically orientated and attempt to conduct homeopathic trials attempting to demonstrate homeopathy's efficacy but these are often of poor quality. A third group argue that by engaging with research and questioning rigorously the false emphasis of the evidence hierarchy, homeopathy and homeopaths will be able to be accepted into an academic world on their own terms with their own methods validated and appreciated. Moreover, the other health and complementary health professionals are asked to provide evidence for what they do. Homeopaths are not a breed apart. The steps of a) asking a question, b) searching for evidence to answer it, c) critically appraising the evidence, d) integrating the evidence into clinical practice, e) evaluating how the steps from a - d went, (Hoffmann 2010) is actually not that demanding.

Research

Research is therefore at the centre of the upgrade from the traditional homeopathic qualification, which was the diploma or advanced diploma, to a degree in complementary medicine and especially homeopathic medicine. These degree courses or masters programs, now place homeopathy within the context of the overall history of healing. From Galen through to Vesalius, from Freud through to the world of evidence-based medicine, a homeopathic degree now emphasizes critical reflection, evaluation and analysis. Questioning and reflecting, criticizing and arguing about the things taught in natural medicine colleges is essentially saying to students, 'Don't believe everything that is told to you, validate it. Think about it. Reflect on it. Is it right? Is it congruent?' What we see is that students coming out of these programs are smart, they don't accept anything just because it's been told to them by someone with a reputation. Students are encouraged to not project impossible qualities onto their lecturers. The cult of the guru, that has infected the profession of homeopathy and continues to do so is discouraged. In the attempt to create a generation of homeopaths with new skills to research and critically think, they are able to take their seat beside practitioners from multiple other modalities. Degrees are not just extra unnecessary classes. Too often degrees have been clip-on's to courses and they involve beefing up medical sciences and irrelevant subjects that others want to see. What is needed is a cogent, coherent, upward spiral of learning grounded in reality.

Thus these seven books are an attempt to raise the bar, ground homeopathic education, encourage debate, critical reflection and research. They are also orientated to professional homeopaths to reflect on what they do, what they learned, what underlying assumptions they carry, where indolence and laziness are a feature of their working lives and maintain their professional development where ever they are. They are also pitched to naturopathic and medical students of homeopathy to fill important practical and conceptual gaps as they wrestle with competing paradigms. When I learnt homeopathy I thought what I was learning was homeopathy. What I now know is that I was being taught a style of homeopathy underpinned by a number of philosophical points of view and assumptions. This is to not say that these assumptions are wrong or that style homeopathy was wrong. It seems to me therefore that it is important to realise that different styles of case taking relate to different ways of practising homeopathy and it is important to understand where one comes from to follow best practice. Flexibility in moving from one style of homeopathy and one style of case taking relevant to that style of homeopathy, is a necessary professional reality depending on where and how one is prescribing. What is crucial is questioning, becoming familiar with and understanding the underpinning assumptions, the sacred cows that go with whatever style of practice one chooses.

Alastair Gray

Philadelphia, USA, 2018

Acknowledgements

Many thanks are warranted in the writing and pulling together this book *Case Management in Homeopathic Medicine* and the companion book *Realities of Contemporary Homeopathy Practice*. Some relate to the homeopathic community and some from further afield.

The first is the editorial work from Helen Vuletin. She provided excellent support, expertise, suggestions, demands and admonition when it was necessary. A sincere debt of gratitude to her for her time and the effort she put into this task. Further, Francis Treuherz in London gave generously of his time, his wealth of knowledge and perspective. Hugely appreciated.

Over the years I've learned much from my Sydney based colleagues, Ken D'Aran, Peter Tumminello, David Levy, Carmen Nicotra who contributed to my understanding of case and people management. Their conversations have in a real way shaped this book. I miss you all.

Thanks to my wife, Denise Straiges, for your uncompromising, inquisitive and rigorous focus on this field and the inspiration you have given me, and restoring my love for homeopathy and encouraging me to revisit this work seven years on.

But it is my clients and patients that have been the real teachers here. I often reflect that my practice has involved a lot of practising. Their patience has enabled me to gain greater clarity and understanding.

Publisher's Note

Case Management is third book in the series titled *"The Landscape of Homeopathic Medicine"*.

The series has been planned keeping in mind the questions which arise in student's and practitioner's minds in regard to different subjects related to homeopathy. This series main intention is to reduce the confusions and publish a number of texts which answer these queries. The books brought out in this series cover different subjects, covering what has been said from the time of Dr Hahnemann to the present day and further, give an analysis from the author and different prominent researchers who have significant experience on the subject.

Case Management explores many different aspects of practice which need to be addressed in the management of cases. This includes the management of the patient as a person, their suffering and other aspects related to a homeopathic practice such as remedy response. The book is a must read for all practitoners to know in which boat they are travelling and how they can really take their practice to a new and better level. This is one subject which is touched on less often in homeopathy, but is nevertheless a very important concern. Were homeopaths to take care of the concerns raised in this book and work on all areas Alastair has discussed, they would benefit from the results in their practices and also help patients know more about the science they have chosen for their treatment.

We wish all readers more success in their clinical practice in times to come.

B. Jain Publishers Pvt. Ltd

Contents

Foreword   *iii*
Introduction to the Series   *vii*
Acknowledgements   *xxi*
Publisher's Note   *xxiii*

Chapters

Part One
Introduction

1. **Introduction**   5
   - 1.1 Management of Cases and People   5
   - 1.2 The Structure of This Book   6
   - 1.3 Why This Book – Reflections and Observations   7
     - 1.3.1 Realities of Practice   8
     - 1.3.2 My Experience   10
     - 1.3.3 My Research   11
       - 1.3.3.1 Some Examples   13
       - 1.3.3.2 The Consequences of 93% and Mixing Modalities   15
       - 1.3.3.3 Impact on Education of Mixed Modalities   15

		1.3.3.4 Limitations of Teaching from Cured Cases	17
		1.3.3.5 Guidance from Our Traditional Literature on Mixing Modalities	18
		1.3.3.6 Measurement Tools	20
	1.3.4	Complex Cases	21
1.4	Homeopathic Medicine and Managing People	22
	1.4.1	Management and Leadership	23
	1.4.2	Identifying Who You Are / Relying on What You Know / Recognising your Default Settings	24
	1.4.3	Management Style	26
	1.4.4	The Need for Management Principles	28
		1.4.4.1 Patience as a Fundamental Principle	29
		1.4.4.2 Highlighting Patience as a Repeatable Principle	30
1.5	The Traditional Emphasis in Homeopathy	31
	1.5.1	What has Case Management Meant?	32
	1.5.2	New Directions	33
1.6	How Hahnemann Managed Cases	35
	1.6.1	House Calls	35
	1.6.2	Virtual Consultations	36
	1.6.3	Compliance	37
	1.6.4	Hahnemann and Money	39
1.7	Remedy versus Person in Relationship	41
	1.7.1	But Where Is the Patient in All of This?	42
1.8	Other Literature	46
1.9	Conclusion	47

Part Two
Getting Busy | Traditional Case Management Strategies, Principles and Techniques

2. **Foundations** — 59
   - 2.1 Introduction — 59
   - 2.2 Follow-up Case Taking — 63
   - 2.3 Structure and Bedrock — 67
   - 2.4 The Basics | Hahnemann's Classification of Disease — 67
   - 2.5 What is an Aggravation? — 71
   - 2.6 What is a Proving Symptom? — 73
   - 2.7 What is a Return of an Old Symptom? — 73
   - 2.8 What is a New Symptom? — 74

3. **History** — 79
   - 3.1 Evaluation of the Patient's Response — 79
   - 3.2 History of the Editions of the *Organon* — 82

4. **Principles** — 87
   - 4.1 The Second Prescription — 87
     - 4.1.1 Hahnemann — 87
     - 4.1.2 Roberts — 88
     - 4.1.3 Chatterjee — 95
     - 4.1.4 Kent: The Second Prescription — 105
     - 4.1.5 Kent: What the People Should Know — 117

5. **Observe, Understand and Act** — 127
   - 5.1 Remedy Reactions — 127
     - 5.1.1 Hahnemann — 127
     - 5.1.2 Roberts — 132

5.1.3 Kent Prognosis after Observing the
Action of the Remedy ... 137

6. Specific Techniques ... 163
6.1 When This Happens ... Do That ... 163
    6.1.1 Sherr ... 163
    6.1.2 Vithoulkas ... 167
    6.1.3 Henriques ... 167
    6.1.4 De Schepper ... 168
    6.1.5 Summary and Collective Wisdom ... 168

7. Repetition of the Dose ... 171
7.1 4th edition of the *Organon* – Opinions ... 171
    7.1.1 Hussey ... 171
    7.1.2 Close ... 178
    7.1.3 Banerjee: The First Prescription ... 182
    7.1.4 Banerjee: The Second Prescription ... 192
    7.1.5 Close Again ... 200

8. The Rich Landscape of Posology ... 213
8.1 Hahnemann's Timeline in the development
and use of the 50 millesimal potencies ... 213
8.2 Critical Thinking ... 214

9. Best Practice, Potency and Administration ... 255
9.1 The Luck of the Draw ... 255
9.2 Burnett on Potency ... 256
9.3 Kent's Flexibility and the Endless Field ... 257
9.4 Hahnemann's Flexibility ... 265
9.5 Little's Best Practice ... 279
9.6 Lippe ... 282

Conclusion Case Management ... 293
References ... 297

Part One
Introduction

Chapter 1

Introduction

Part One | Contents

1.1 Management of Cases and People
1.2 The Structure of This Book
1.3 Why This Book - Reflections and Observations
    1.3.1 Realities of Practice
    1.3.2 My Experience
    1.3.3 My Research
    1.3.4 Complex Cases
1.4 Homeopathic Medicine and Managing People
    1.4.1 Management and Leadership
    1.4.2 Identifying Who You Are / Relying on What You Know / Recognising Your Default Settings
    1.4.3 Management Style
    1.4.4 The Need for Management Principles
1.5 The Traditional Emphasis in Homeopathy
    1.5.1 What has Case Management Meant?
    1.5.2 New Directions
1.6 How Hahnemann Managed Cases
    1.6.1 House calls
    1.6.2 Virtual Consultations

- 1.6.3 Compliance
- 1.6.4 Hahnemann and Money
- 1.7 Remedy versus Person in Relationship
  - 1.7.1 But Where Is the Patient in All of This?
- 1.8 Other Literature
- 1.9 Conclusion

Chapter 1
Introduction

1.1 Management of Cases and People

This book has nothing to do with choosing the medicine. The emphasis on finding the right remedy, the perfect medicine is so often stressed in homeopathy, during homeopathic conversations, in homeopathic classrooms and consultation rooms. This book does not deal with that issue at all. This book does not deal with the *similar* in any way, or even the close similar remedy. In fact there are two books dealing with aspects of case management here to be read in tandem. They are volumes III and IV in the *Landscape of Homeopathic Medicine* series. The first, this one focuses on tradition and best practice over 200 years, while the second focuses on contemporary and complex patient case management. They are very different, but they go together. Neither this book or its sister have anything to do with the right remedy.

A much more important topic is addressed here - people. This book, *Case Management in Homeopathic Medicine*, and its companion, *Realities of Contemporary Homeopathy Practice* are person focused and they discuss how as health practitioners in the 21st century, we can utilise the instructions from the giants of our profession who lived in other times to maximise the results of our work, how to manage our cases well and expertly to optimise results.

Implicit in this work is the idea that there is as much value in managing people, placing the person being treated at the very centre of the process, as opposed to the practitioner, remedy, or the therapeutics. This is the time to maximise your skills of creating rapport over and above your skills of being a detective, finding the disease, the totality of symptoms and the characteristics, a time to go beyond the complete symptom and find the best match, the most similar remedy.

These books also explore how, through modifying our own behaviours, through engaging in a discussion about establishing principles, we can encourage our patients to comply, to follow instructions and to maximise the impact of the medicine that they have taken. These are therefore books about being able to identify what has happened, and make a clear decision about what to do next.

1.2 The Structure of This Book

This work, Vol III *Landscape of Homeopathic Medicine Series* on exploring issues of Case Management is divided into two distinct parts:

Part One | Introduction

This section provides context around the issue of case management, why it's important, what we have been doing as a profession for the last 200 years, and future directions.

Part Two | Getting Busy | Traditional Case Management Strategies, Principles and Techniques

This section provides context and commentary on all the traditional case management strategies adopted by homeopaths and articulated by authors since the beginnings of the profession in the early 1800's. The traditional literature is to be found in books, articles and texts all over the place and never in a one-stop shop. This book addresses this obstacle. Just who said what about remedy reactions, repeating the remedy, overcoming obstacles to cure, the second prescription? There is also advice from the masters from Hahnemann to Kent, Chatterjee, Roberts and Close, as well as a commentary on how useful that advice might be for us in these times.

Volume IV in the *Landscape of Homeopathic Medicine Series, Realities of Contemporary Homeopathy Practice* is very different. While part two looks at the literature and is more academic in tone, the next book represents the author's opinion. This section provides context, commentary and principles of being a homeopath in the pragmatic reality of today. It builds a case around the need for contemporary clinical principles, and highlights the context within which we are practicing, and charts a path forward.

1.3 Why This Book – Reflections and Observations

After innumerable conversations with practitioners, students, graduates, and onlookers, there is enough evidence to suggest that:

- Contemporary homeopaths are often not prepared for the realities of practice

- Experience gained in the classroom is not congruent with running a modern practice
- Research is paramount to ensuring that our profession continues to thrive, and homeopaths must conduct research in their own practices in the form of a clinical audit
- There is an increase in frequency of complex cases, typically as a result of complications from conventional drugs, as well as homeopathic medicines, and lifestyle choices

As a consequence, we need to establish clear principles of working.

What is it like to be a homeopath in the early 2000s? Usually this discussion happens at conferences at lunch-time, but rarely in the classroom during college. It's a bit like acting. Actors go to acting school to learn to be actors. They learn techniques and methods and strategies. Yet no one talks to them about what it's like to be an actor. And it's hard. There's a continuous cycle of audition, rejection, audition, rejection.

1.3.1 Realities of Practice

Everyone loves a story and a description of reality, an analogy. Sometimes a direct approach leads to trouble. It can be too confrontational. As Emily Dickenson says in her magnificent poem, *Tell All The Truth:*

> *Tell all the truth but tell it slant,*
> *Success in circuit lies,*
> *Too bright for our infirm delight*
> *The truth's superb surprise*
> *As lightning to the children eased*
> *With explanation kind,*

Introduction

The truth must dazzle gradually
Or every man be blind.

Over the years, I have struggled to find metaphors or ways of describing homeopathy. It's unfortunate therefore that the best metaphor for the reality of homeopathy practice happens to be a sporting one. As a golfer, you have a set of tools, clubs and you have an intention to get the ball in the hole. As a homeopath, your tools include a repertory, textbooks, proving books. The patient is represented by the ball. Your aim is always to get the client to the result, which is health in the shortest amount of time, in as few shots as possible gently, rapidly, and permanently. There is always the promise of the hole-in-one, which may actually happen statistically 1% of the time in the reality of daily practice. The chances of it really happening are minimal.

The reality of practice is that we get close, and we work with partial similars and we do our best. This reality still emphasises the medicine, and the correct remedy. So in this book, the emphasis is shifted. We focus on Hahnemann's instructions for curing one-sided cases, dealing with aggravations, and dealing with the return of old symptoms. Rarely do we achieve brilliant prescriptions. Rarely do we hit holes in one. In reality, we do our best.

It didn't take long in my own homeopathic practice to realise that much of what I learned, just like a lawyer or an accountant I suppose, was theoretical and not always accurate. Perhaps it was also that I moved countries. The types of clients seen in one country were not the types of clients that I was seeing in another. What I call the realities of practice were a sharp awakening for me. No one taught me this at college.

Often I had no hope of understanding the complexity of their pathology. Strangely, they did what they wanted as well. They took what they wanted, they ignored my instructions, and often were not as committed to their health as I was. Patients had different expectations, and most confusing of all, they went to seek advice from elsewhere, often at the same time as they were seeking advice from me. This last point left me bewildered. Did my patients simply have no idea? Surely they would soon realise that by taking other medicine, or seeing some other practitioner, they were compromising the possibility of getting the best results with my medicine. On many occasions, I found myself feeling frustrated, unappreciated, misunderstood, and not knowing what to do.

1.3.2 My Experience

We are all influenced by what happens to us. Principle and direction are shaped by the filter of our experience, which of course is the coalface of our clinical practices. A lot of the ideas that I'm presenting here come from my interactions with a number of very specific clients. I am not referring to the clients that come in and talk, get the remedy and take it, and then go home. When I talk about specific clients, I am talking about the ones that want to take you home to dinner to introduce you to their daughter. It comes from having clients who have 21st century lifestyles that I can't even begin to articulate on paper. It comes from having the wildest conversations with patients. It comes from treating people with massively complex multi-miasmatic diseases. It comes from having expectations of what a day in the life of a contemporary homeopath should look like, and what it actually does end up looking like. It comes from getting hammered in the media constantly in the last six years. And my experience comes from research.

Introduction

Lastly, it certainly comes from clients that didn't get better after my treatment.

1.3.3 My Research

I come from an eclectic place when it comes to the teaching and learning of homeopathic medicine. Originally from New Zealand, I did my formative years there, and amongst other things studied law and history. Surprisingly, both have come into a significant amount use in my homeopathic practice, and in my years teaching and lecturing about homeopathic medicine, and more recently managing a department in a private university.

From the outset, when I discovered homeopathy and began to study, I was fascinated by research. Early on in the process, I discovered provings, and to this day am still passionate about this aspect of our art and science. In terms of other passions, the ingredients of thriving practice and the treatment of male patients, were then and still are, areas of particular interest to me. Being heavily influenced by a Masters of Science that I undertook in 2006, a new emphasis grew within me on the necessity to apply the rigour of evidence, critical thinking and critical evaluation to my homeopathy. In addition, I'm endlessly fascinated by new technologies and how they augment or detract from learning and practice, and how they can be used in the practice and teaching of homeopathic medicine.

It's my understanding that all homeopaths, everywhere, have always been researchers. People wrongly assume that research is about statistics and having a Ph.D. It can be that, but usually it is not. In practice, homeopaths can do excellent, simple clinical audits, and other meaningful pieces of research. A number of years ago I conducted a clinical audit of my practice that took me about a week. It was in the summer and I didn't do much else that week. I just audited my practice. And it was around the 15-year mark I had been in practice, I call it *Alastair's 15-year clinical audit*. I noticed that I was getting a lot of clients. I realised they were telling me many similar things. I noticed that my results were okay. What I really noticed was that they liked talking to me. I was also clearly getting results, and not necessarily because of the remedies prescribed. I was getting results because of the questions I was asking, and perhaps, ultimately because of me.

For better or worse, I noticed in the process of this audit that a lot of my prescribing had moved from being based on broad totality prescriptions, as I had learnt in college, to being more orientated to organ prescribing, affinity, and location. I was often prescribing on keynotes, or my knowledge of therapeutics. I started to learn more from the naturopath or the herbalist down the corridor in the clinic, and started to think about what they were doing with their clients. Whenever we shared clients, I was thinking about and talking to them about their interventions. I had long since dropped the idea of suppression. I was always busy. I was doing smaller totality prescriptions.

This clinical audit coincided with the first year of my masters program. In that program, I was asked to do a piece of research so the two projects became one. My audit and research revealed that a surprising amount of my clients were getting multiple interventions. They were coming to see me as well as seeing a chiropractor, the pharmacist, doing Pilates, doing yoga, taking their fish oils, and getting a weekly massage. There were multiple interventions and they were coming from multiple modalities.

Introduction

On interviewing some of my clients in a gentle informal piece of research, I discovered that they were simply doing what they wanted to. They absolutely saw me as part of their team. So it was a surprise to learn that 93% of my clients were 'behaving badly'. Our (my) patients were no longer seeing us as they did 200 or 100 or even 10 years ago. They are doing lots of other stuff. When I say that they're behaving badly, I have my tongue in my cheek. Of course they're just doing what they want to. In my last 500 cases, 93% were getting treatment from another practitioner, and taking other medicines in addition to mine.

1.3.3.1 Some Examples

A man came to see me in 2007. He wanted me to help him lose weight. He also had a furuncle. It was the size of his fist. The furuncle was located in his groin. It was complicated. He was 140 kilos. Enormous. He loved exercise but he couldn't do any. Why? Because when he sweated, he got terrible itches and rashes and an eruption in his groin. Even swimming aggravated his skin, his furuncle, his mood and depression. In addition to these physical symptoms, he had spent the last three months in a private psychiatric hospital. It was very expensive and very exclusive. He was getting daily psychological help. What would you do? Where would you start? Oh, did I mention that he was also on the following medications:

Epilim 2500	*Anti inflammatories*
Parnate 60	*Nurofen plus*
Lipitor 40	*Roaccutane*
Seroquel 750	*Effexor 375*
Levoxyl for the thyroid 100	*Valium 10....*
Metabolism meds	

And it is not just allopathic medicines making our jobs all the more complex. What about those patients already on homeopathic remedies?

Case of pre-menstrual syndrome. The patient was also on the following homeopathic medicines:

Ferr, hyper, berberis, sepia, ars, nicotiana, merc viv, arg nit, mosch, e-coli and ovary co.

Case ADHD. The patient was also on the following supplements and homeopathic medicines:

Acetylcholine chloride, Dopamine, Epinephrine, Gallic Acid, Gamma-amino-butyric acid, Histamine, Insulin, L-Dopa, Malvin, Melatonin, Noreinephrine, Salsolinol, Seratonin, Taurine, Tyramine in 6, 12, 30, 200x, 12, 30, 200c, Cobalt, Copper, Gelseminum, Iodine, Vanadium 12x, Ginko, Gotu kola, Hydrastis, Lomatium, Panax, Tarax 6x

In my clinical audit, it was typical for the patient presenting with herpes to also be seeing a Chinese medicine doctor and taking Valtrex. The person with obesity was also at the gym, working with Weight Watchers and taking supplements. The teenager with acne was also taking a range of skin products through a naturopath. The patient with lymphoma was also getting chemotherapy, was seeing a psychotherapist, and getting bodywork. The client with infertility was seeing a therapist, and getting IVF as well seeing me. The patient with cancer was getting therapy, homeopathy, nutrition, energetic bodywork, chemotherapy, seeing an oncologist, a Chinese herbal medicine practitioner and getting acupuncture.

Ironically, the patient with an unidentified ulcerous skin condition was getting no other treatment at all and only coming to see me. He was a recently arrived refugee from Pakistan, and had been getting homeopathic treatment all of his life.

1.3.3.2 The Consequences of 93% and Mixing Modalities

On reflection what does this 93% mean? That 93% is my statistic in my practice. Of course on talking to many other homeopathic practitioners over the years, I've noticed that they have their own statistics. Some homeopaths quote having a statistic around the same mark, some much lower, and a few higher. Nevertheless it's an important point. I am not the only one that has noticed this trend in homeopathic medicine over the last five years or so. From India to Brazil, to the USA to Australia, patients are mixing modalities and getting multiple interventions at the same time. I know for sure that from my last clinical audit, 93% of my clients were mixing modalities, and as a consequence perceive me as part of their team of healthcare practitioners. A practitioner in California told me 95% of her clients were getting chiropractic, massage, acupuncture or herbs. Another practitioner told me 100% of her clients were getting some kind of other treatment in addition to homeopathy. What are the implications and the consequences? This mixing of modalities has significant impact on our claims about cure and about how we approach education.

1.3.3.3 Impact on Education of Mixed Modalities

One of the obvious impacts of this simple statistic is that it is at odds with how we teach homeopathy. To a huge extent, we still teach homeopathy as if it's the only intervention going into a patient at any one time. We teach homeopathy as a stand-alone discipline. Though it is clearly not, especially in the Western world. In medical and professional homeopathy, patients are absolutely seeing multiple practitioners and getting multiple interventions; they are getting the kitchen sink thrown at their condition.

Yet still in classrooms, we teach case management, case taking, as if homeopathic treatment is the only thing that the patient will be getting. I have serious reservations about the pragmatic value of this approach now. In other words, it's not real. What can students expect in practice from their clients? What are patients assuming and thinking? What does integration actually mean? In some parts of the world, integrative medicine is a dirty word. In some places, 'integrative' means conventional medicine stealing the best of complementary medicine. In other parts of the world, the word 'integrated' is preferred.

The traditional emphasis on homeopathy has always been about the remedy. Hahnemann said it, Kent said it, Margaret Tyler said it. The emphasis is on getting it right. In addition to that, in the 20th century and now in the 21st century, there is also an obsession with getting to the centre of the problem. A confluence of post-Jungian ideas have been borrowed and have become part of the fabric of contemporary homeopathy, under the influence of Whitmont, Vithoulkas, Schmidt, Scholten and Sankaran, and these have meant that this seductive idea is now pervasive across the profession. Yet it never started in that way. Never in the minds of Hahnemann and Bönninghausen, as we understand it through their writings, was there such a strong emphasis on perfection, and finding the right remedy. The practice of homeopathy from the outset was using multiple remedies prescribed after multiple conversations.

As an educationalist, we see students doing some strange things with this emphasis on the right remedy, and going for the centre. At a certain point in the training, they freak out, they lose confidence, they ask a question that should never be asked and that is, 'can I possibly do this?'

1.3.3.4 Limitations of Teaching from Cured Cases

Simple research skills utterly changed my practice. As a direct result, these skills have made me talk about homeopathy differently. As a direct result, they have also highlighted the absolute limitations and perils of learning from case studies.

Recently I was teaching in India. I was explaining to the class why there is such significant opposition from the scientific and clinical researching communities about teaching a medical modality from the perspective of 'cured cases'. I was demonstrating that there is too much bias, too many other possible interfering factors that can get in the way before we can say for sure, 'this remedy cured that case'. I was making the point as gently as I could. I was startled when, at the break, an Indian doctor approached me and chastised me for not showing more of my cases.

World-wide, homeopaths still teach homeopathy from cured cases. I've done it so many times myself. I have a patient to whom I've given *Scorpion*, and the patient has an amazing response. I write it up and publish it as my *Scorpion* case. I have a patient that responds well to *Germanium*. I write it up. Our industry journals are full of cured cases. Participants at seminars demand it also. We need to remind ourselves that this evidence constitutes low-level evidence in the biomedical world. It's not that we should stop doing it by any means. In addition, we need to have a conversation about how to do it well, with congruence and integrity.

1.3.3.5 Guidance from Our Traditional Literature on Mixing Modalities

While emphasising case management strongly in his writings, Hahnemann's guidelines on patients seeking other treatments are pretty thin. While talking about mesmerism, bathing and a couple of other interventions in the *Organon of Medicine*, there is not much else. Treuherz (2010) clearly shows that Hahnemann's patients were getting all sorts of 'other' treatments from him; electricity, nutritional advice, lifestyle advice. Eating asparagus while lying in bed, reading licentious books, and having voluptuous thoughts was clearly not okay.

Footnote to § 260: Coffee; fine Chinese and other herb teas; beer prepared with medicinal vegetable substances unsuitable for the patient's state; so-called fine liquors made with medicinal spices; all kinds of punch; spiced chocolate; odorous waters and perfumes of many kinds; strong-scented flowers in the apartment; tooth powders and essences and perfumed sachets compounded of drugs; highly spiced dishes and sauces; spiced cakes and ices; crude medicinal vegetables for soups; dishes of herbs, roots and stalks of plants possessing medicinal qualities; asparagus with long green tips, hops, and all vegetables possessing medicinal properties, celery, onions; old cheese, and meats that are in a state of decomposition, or that passes medicinal properties (as the flesh and fat of pork, ducks and geese, or veal that is too young and sour viands), ought just as certainly to be kept from patients as they should avoid all excesses in food, and in the use of sugar and salt, as also spirituous drinks, undiluted with water, heated rooms, woollen clothing next the skin, a sedentary life in close apartments, or the frequent indulgence in mere passive exercise (such as riding, driving or swinging), prolonged suckling, taking a long siesta in a recumbent posture in bed, sitting up long at night, uncleanliness, unnatural debauchery, enervation by

Introduction

reading obscene books, reading while lying down, Onanism or imperfect or suppressed intercourse in order to prevent conception, subjects of anger, grief or vexation, a passion for play, over-exertion of the mind or body, especially after meals, dwelling in marshy districts, damp rooms, penurious living, etc. All these things must be as far as possible avoided or removed, in order that the cure may not be obstructed or rendered impossible. Some of my disciples seem needlessly to increase the difficulties of the patient's dietary by forbidding the use of many more, tolerably indifferent things, which is not to be commended.

Over the years, we've received directives from many other writers and sources. Stuart Close (1924), Vithoulkas (1980), Bill Gray (2012) and Linda Johnston (2012) have given clear guidelines on what patients can and can't do, should and should not do when they are getting treatment. In fact, some give a bewildering array of lifestyle changes that must happen and substances that have to be avoided before commencing any homeopathic treatment.

Trawling through the literature, I could find only one example of a contemporary book that spoke about this aspect of multiple interventions:

Management. Many of our patients are already seeing a body worker or physician (chiropractor, osteopath) when they begin homeopathic treatment. Also, these health professionals often refer to us in an attempt to keep their patients away from the risks of allopathic medications or surgery. Startlingly, some homeopaths, out of fear of antidoting, ask such referred patients to refrain from seeing their referring practitioner. Needless to say, this practice is divisive in the alternative community and does more harm than good. Instead we must work with our alternative colleagues and discuss our concerns rather than put our patients in a position of divided loyalty (Morrison 1998).

Beyond the preceding passage, there is nothing further in the modern academic literature or contemporary homeopathic literature on this obvious issue. Worse, when it comes to published cases, I could only find one published case (Rothenberg *Simillimum* 2005), that talked about other interventions being used as well as the homeopathic one. I simply cannot believe that is real, given what we know about modern patient behaviour.

When I question practitioners about how they deal with this issue, these are the types of answers I get:

- *Deal with it*
- *Do your best*
- *Muddle on through*
- *Make it up*
- *Get over it*
- *Somehow work out what is the medicine and what is the other stuff*
- *Determine what proportion of the result is due to the therapeutic relationship and what is the remedy*

1.3.3.6 Measurement Tools

There is a further consequence. Most homeopaths don't measure their results. Some don't bother, some don't know how to, some are too busy and they see the client out and move to the next one. This omission has profound effects for us as a broader profession. Of course, there are multiple measurement tools in medicine. One of the best that is simple and easy to use is MYMOP, which stands for Measure Yourself Medical Outcome Profile (questionnaire). It is now widely used in complementary medicine. It is a simple process of measuring the presenting symptom or symptoms. It measures patient satisfaction. It can be used to examine cost benefit also. Consistent use of an agreed audit tool would go a huge way to creating statistical facts about our clinical effectiveness. The measurement tool used must be comprehensive enough and robust enough to take into account and reflect multiple interventions. In other words, was the result achieved through:

- Just homeopathy
- Homeopathy and one modality
- Homeopathy and many modalities

The use of MYMOP has met some considerable success around the world as an accurate measurement tool. Further initiatives such as training homeopaths and students to learn how to write up and publish cases correctly would go a long way.

1.3.4 Complex Cases

The other reason for a need to discuss management strategies is that our cases are getting harder. I've been travelling to many parts of the world teaching about treating complex and difficult cases and uncompliant people for many years. It started by being asked to teach a one-hour class to undergraduate students in New Zealand. I remember my original reaction, which was, 'it doesn't make any sense'. Because we individualise, we just treat people so it doesn't matter who they are or what they have. There is no such thing as difficult patients that would only ever come into consideration. That's what I believed then. I gave a lecture anyway and it was well received. It got me to thinking.

Soon afterwards, by some piece of synchronicity, I was asked to restructure a whole subject at an undergraduate college. The curriculum being taught was not meeting the professional or educational standards and needed a rewrite. There were four areas where I had experienced considerable difficulty in my own practice. The following broad categories of patients indicate where things have either gone slowly or not at all:

- Anxious patients are easily the most complex group of clients that I've ever had in my practice
- Patients with a compulsive relationship to alcohol or recreational drugs
- Patients that are heavily reliant on medical drugs
- Patients with eating disorders

1.4 Homeopathic Medicine and Managing People

What does management mean? What does it mean to manage someone? How do you manage somebody? If you're not occupying a management position at work, then you are surely managing your patients, your kids, your husband, your finances or your studies. But I don't remember receiving any instruction about the subject at all. Ever.

Homeopaths have come from all sorts of different backgrounds. Over the years I've met homeopaths who are also geologists, historians, hippies, dropouts, school teachers and all sorts of other areas in between. Our profession is rich in diversity. It's rare however when homeopaths have come from a corporate environment where they've been involved in the formal management of people. But that does not matter so much because managing people can take all forms and shapes. Often I have heard homeopathic students say, 'I'm just a mum.' But in fact they may well have as good, if not better management skills, than anyone else because of the Herculean task of raising children. Managing cases and managing people is all about identifying your own capacities and predilections first.

1.4.1 Management and Leadership

These are obviously different things. Leaders lead. Managers manage. Leaders inspire. Managers implement. Leaders create strategy. Managers deliver that strategy.

While there are differences, the two roles also have a considerable amount of overlap. Over the years while travelling and teaching homeopathy, I have asked students and practitioners to identify their role models for management style. There is a surprising array of heartfelt answers given, including the Dalai Lama, Rajan Sankaran, Eckhart Tolle, Genghis Khan, Elderly quaker ladies, My mother, My kids, Mahatma Gandhi, and Martin Luther King.

> 'Their leadership style was based upon having a vision, a goal inspiring people to share their vision through excellent communication skills responding with steadfastness and the vision of other's behaviour choices of which they sometimes did not approve. We can extrapolate this into practice, that is not backing down on goal that is set even when the client makes excuses not to hold onto it, using good indication of persuasive skills to bring them back to that vision'

Many homeopaths are inspired by Hahnemann, and many are inspired by John Lennon, or those who've overcome life challenges and came out the other side.

I think that in the study of homeopathy these are useful conversations to have and reflections to consider. At the end of the day, leadership and management is easy when there is plain sailing, when the sails are full of wind and the crew have full bellies. Leadership and management skills come to the fore in homeopathic practice when things are *not* going well, when the crew are hungry, when you're lost, when you're under attack. Having clear leadership and a strong management model to assist you and your clients through these difficult times is very important. It is vitally important then to ask the questions: who inspires me, how did they lead, and how did they manage in times of trial.

1.4.2 Identifying Who You Are / Relying on What You Know / Recognising your Default Settings

Recently I was asked to teach a webinar series. I was amazed when I read the backgrounds of the participants. All of them were homeopaths and a couple were homeopathic students. Some came from Canada, some from Australia, the UK, the USA, Mexico, Italy, New Zealand, Hong Kong, and Thailand. Even more extraordinary was where those people came from before they found homeopathy. There is a richness in our community. It's really only in India at the moment, and a few other countries around the world, where we have young people coming from high school directly into homeopathic training. In other words, in India there is no shortage of 18-year-olds wanting to study homeopathy. But most other parts of the world, we get a different demographic. We find people wanting a change. We find people on their second or even third careers. In this webinar series, I had a former accountant, a teacher, an aircraft engineer, someone in automobile recycling, an airline pilot, retail and office management consultants for small businesses, an analytical chemist, a consultant in environmental consulting, an interpreter, a nurse, a beautician, someone with a business degree, someone in video postproduction, marketing, advertising and public relations, mothers, wives, boyfriends, husbands. I encouraged all these participants to identify their leadership style, their management style and the skills they bought with them to homeopathic medicine. Whether we know it or not, we are constantly managing people and situations. When we manage our patients, we are generally doing nothing other than falling back on the default settings of what we already know.

Over the years, I've adopted all sorts of strategies to assist people with getting to where they want and where I want them to get to. I recognise for example, in my personal, not professional life that I yell. Somehow, still in some dark recess, is a part of me that will have a tantrum if I don't get what I want. I'm also a sulker. Somehow I developed that strategy survival at a young age to let everyone around me know that I wasn't happy. I just sat on my cold anger in a position of perverse power and made everyone's life miserable. These days, I have developed other strategies because I have other responsibilities. With my team at Endeavour College I've used all sorts of strategies from silence to insults, to ignoring, to pleading, to desperation, to tears, to rewarding with flowers and chocolate, and threatening the sack and instant dismissal.

None of them worked at all. Here's what I have learned doesn't work for me:

- Sulking
- Bullying
- Rewarding, which essentially boils down to bribery
- Passive-aggressive behaviour
- Threatening
- Pretending to be Mussolini

Here is what does work. People respond to being part of the vision. People engage with projects and pull on their oar, and do their part, and take it for the team, when they buy in to a vision and direction. They must be connected to the vision. This is how Shackleton, Steve Waugh, Montgomery, Ritchie McCaw and Churchill lead their people towards a desired direction. Leadership is the most amazing thing. Some lead from the front. Some inspire. Some are first up the ladder and over the wall and out of the trench. We employ all of these techniques and strategies daily with our patients.

1.4.3 Management Style

Previously I was horrified by the idea of management. I thought that management is what all of the people that failed on all the other subjects ended up doing. Ironically, these days they all seem to earn five times more money than I do however. Having some clarity on the type of risk taker that you are really assists in the practice of homeopathy. Identifying your own management style is very important, and the earlier that happens in the development of your practice the better. And it can be a steep learning curve. For example, it took me many, many years in practice before I was able to say 'no' to a client. It took me many years in practice before I realised that I carry a projection of authority, and that it is entirely appropriate and expected that sometimes I give clear direction. 'Don't do this behaviour, It is making you sick,' for example. 'No you can't expect me to be available for you when you want me to.' 'I understand that you have needs but this is also Christmas day.' The constant reflective question to homeopaths is, 'How do you manage a situation? What do you do?'

Again, in questioning homeopathic students and practitioners worldwide about their management style, the way they manage their clients in stressful situations, the way they manage people, the way they get their clients on board with them, there have been wide array of responses.

1.	'My management style is casual and adaptable. My patients tend to look up to me.'
2.	'My management style is mostly relationship orientated. I try to connect with people, understand where they are coming from and educate and ask for their cooperation.'
3.	'I have an interesting style which I've noticed, I ask in a lovely way, and I tell in a lovely way, then a yell, yes apparently in a lovely way, and finally I threaten them.'
4.	'Patient management is all about intensive education. Sometimes the amount of time it can take is overwhelming.'
5.	Patient management for me is like a dance, to do well with somebody you need to firstly be present focused and on balance, try and leave the ego aside, sometimes take the lead from a patient, I try and have fun, the best dances are improvised.'
6.	'I try to create rapport and then gain their trust. I teach and give lots of information. I try to communicate clearly and I have handouts for them on various topics.'
7.	'My management style, my way or the highway.'
8.	'Keep calm and carry on, work with them not against them.'

1.4.4 The Need for Management Principles

Very early on in my practice, I heard Jeremy Sherr say something that changed my mind about what I have been doing. He said something very obvious, that the remedy represented he thought, about 30% of the curative response in a case. 2% at most could be put down to the potency and the rest was about case management. What he meant at that stage was that it is the management of the remedy and the skills of the second prescription that determine how well a homeopathic medicine does for the client.

We are lacking fundamental principles to underpin best practices in homeopathic practice. The basics are already sound and embedded in our clinical work. However, our clients are no longer the same. They are biologically the same as Hahnemann's patients 200 years ago, yet they are different in all other ways. One of the hardest aspects of practising homeopathy is managing the expectations of clients. Many people come to homeopathy cold. They don't really know what to expect. Then homeopaths ask annoying questions. These questions of course are completely legitimate, can be extremely time consuming, and bulk out what might have been a 40-minute consultation to well over an hour. People are not used to this style of consultation. Anxious people ask a lot of questions, 'how do I take the remedy'? 'Is it four or five drops'? 'I read on the internet about toothpaste'. Managing all of these questions and concerns take an extraordinary amount of patience and time on behalf of both the patient and practitioner.

It soon became apparent in my exploration of managing difficult cases that there was very little about this topic in any of the literature. There is certainly some literature about managing difficult cases in other modalities such as physiotherapy, medicine, psychotherapy, and the other specialisations within medicine. These modalities talk about it at length. To me, in homeopathy, this work needs significant improvement, dialogue and debate. It is simply not good enough to make it up as we go along in a profession. For too long, we've been getting away with these informal practices, deluding ourselves to some degree that we are doing anything other than psuedo-science. For the credibility of our profession, we must have principles to work with to underpin clinical decision making.

1.4.4.1 Patience as a Fundamental Principle

Having the ability to wait is a fundamental quality of a thriving homeopath. As Francis Treuherz reminds me, 'How many homeopaths does it take to change a light bulb? Two. One to give the remedy and one to wait.' While it's a great quality to be patient and know when to push, it is also very important to know when to yield and wait. Doubly important is to know when the impatience is coming from your own projection or your own agenda of how the healing should be taking place as opposed to what the patient wants. Again, to paraphrase Jeremy Sherr, homeopathy is the medicine of nothing. You give nothing in the bottle. And then nothing happens. Of course everything happens. Whether it is attributed to a near perfect intervention or not is a completely different matter.

If there is agreement that a fundamental quality, an important psychographic factor, and a basic quality of a thriving homeopath is patience, then it begs the question how can patience be taught if it doesn't come naturally? While I am not sure, I think travelling is a great way to learn it, and looking after other people is another good way. Spending time with your parents for example, or travelling in another country with a different sense of time can assist. Any situation, usually one involving a different culture, teaches us about time, patience and waiting, a bus in India or Ecuador, sitting in a restaurant in Fiji. People have their own exquisite sense of timing and whether or not it bears any relationship to yours is up for grabs. Chances are it won't be.

1.4.4.2 Highlighting Patience as a Repeatable Principle

Although there will be differences in the way individuals execute this principle in practice, this flow chart summarizes the key points of this principle that will lead to the greatest chances of successful implementation, and most importantly can be repeated by all practitioners:

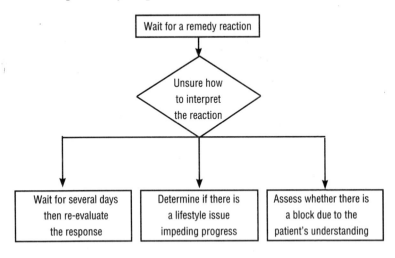

Knowing just what to do in the moment the patient says, 'I've been feeling well for three weeks but in the last few days I think I'm getting worse, can you give me something else'. You might think to ask the question, where are you in your menstrual cycle today, leading to the understanding that this could be a normal premenstrual buildup rather than the remedy not working and requiring a change. This could be evidence that all was going well.	So often in our practices, patients need to make decisions about their marriages, giving up alcohol, moving out from living with their mum.	Wait for patients to move through a barrier to their understanding or a breakthrough in their personal development. Know just what it means when a patient is mentally and emotionally better but the presenting symptom is the same.

1.5 The Traditional Emphasis in Homeopathy

Up until the present, the great textbooks by Stuart Close, Roberts, Kent and Vithoulkas writing on case management have emphasised the usual aspects when it comes to managing cases and people. They have rightly emphasised that a thriving homeopath knows these traditional homeopathic management skills back to front.

1.5.1 What has Case Management Meant?

These are the issues that are addressed in the second part of this book, things such as the second prescription, repetition of the dose, when to act and when to wait. In the past, case management has meant knowing the following:

- Evaluation of the response to the remedy
- Repetition of the dose
- Second prescription rules of Kent, Bönninghausen
- Remedy reactions as articulated by Vithoulkas or Henriques
- Administration issues, such as method of delivery of the medicine; dry dosing versus wet dosing, one pill, 5 drops, split doses, and succussion

For generations, students have learned case management in homeopathy by reading the *Organon* and the other excellent texts. Follow the rules, be unprejudiced, be faithful in tracing the picture of the disease, attention to detail, and accuracy. Case management seems to be best summed up by aphorism three:

> If the physician clearly perceives what is to be cured in diseases, that is to say, in every individual case of disease (knowledge of disease, indication), if he clearly perceives what is curative in medicines, that is to say, in each individual medicine (knowledge of medicinal powers), and if he knows how to adapt, according to clearly defined principles, what is curative in medicines to what he has discovered to be undoubtedly morbid in the patient, so that the recovery must ensue – to adapt it, as well in respect to the suitability of the medicine most appropriate according to its mode of action to the case before him (choice of the remedy,

the medicine indicated), as also in respect to the exact mode of preparation and quantity of it required (proper dose), and the proper period for repeating the dose: - if, finally, *he knows the obstacles to recovery in each case and is aware how to remove them*, so that the restoration may be permanent: then he understands how to treat judiciously and rationally, and he is a true practitioner of the healing art (Hahnemann 1921).

Traditionally, there was a clear emphasis on getting people to change their behaviour and stop behaving badly, which is nicely summed up by Close:

> It is taken for granted that the physician, acting in another capacity than that of a prescriber of homoeopathic medicine, will remove the causes of the disease and the obstacles to cure as far as possible before he addresses himself to the task of selecting and administering the remedy which is homoeopathic to the symptoms of the case, by which the cure is to be performed.
>
> It stands to reason, as Hahnemann says, that every intelligent physician, having a knowledge of rational etiology, will first remove by appropriate means, as far as possible, every exciting and maintaining cause of disease and obstacle to cure, and endeavor to establish a correct and orderly course of living for his patient, with due regard to mental and physical hygiene. Failing to do this, but little impression can be made by homoeopathic remedies, and what slight impression is made will be of short duration (Close 1924).

1.5.2 New Directions

In the 21st century, with contemporary clients, this approach is antiquated and very 'old school'. The significant practical and theoretical work being achieved in the area of drug and alcohol counceling points to other strategies, risk management and harm minimisation. This book will discuss that while there are clear compromises when working with patients that are still living their chosen lifestyles and are not removing those factors that are contributing to their disease, it is a more humanistic approach. As practitioners move forward with their own casework, we can begin to compare more contemporary approaches in the treatment of these clients with the harsher directives of some more Victorian approaches, Close in particular.

Because of my own experiences, research and reflection, it dawned on me slowly over the years that this approach to removing obstacles to cure and maintaining causes, for those clients taking the Pill or having a reliance on some substance, was out of step with the modern world and other close healing modalities. And it slowly dawned on me that in addition to the remedy, other key features that went into the process of assisting a person through their healing was seeing them as a person, engaging in a relationship with them, getting good information out of them that might take time, as well as the remedy.

I didn't really realise at the time that this is considered to be a *humanistic* or a *person-centred approach*. All I really knew was that I had been influenced by my teachers: Misha Norland, Miranda Castro, and later by Ian Townsend, Kate Chatfield, and Jean Duckworth. It involved being with patients as opposed to doing things to them. It involved realising that empathy, congruence, authenticity, unconditional positive regard, and self-disclosure also work as therapeutic tools, not just what Hahnemann said.

At the coalface in my own practice, my homeopathic approach could therefore best be summed up, as an approach using the Hahnemann/Bönninghausen method, KISS method (keep it simple, stupid), person centred, and where appropriate a willingness to aim for the central issues and sensations if they can be perceived.

1.6 How Hahnemann Managed Cases

Many practitioners leave college unprepared for practice, emotionally and practically. Many are still unconfident about their capacity to manage the relationship. Given that what has been said previously differs in approach to traditional homeopathic approaches, it is important to reflect on what we know of case management strategies of the great homeopaths.

Two recent authors in particular, Jütte in his book (2005) and Treuherz (2010) have shed some light on the case management style, strategies and activities of Hahnemann. He did so many of the usual things that any physician at the time would do, and there were also many things that set him apart. We can learn a lot from them.

1.6.1 House Calls

It was clear that Hahnemann did not like house calls. There were of course a few exceptions. House calls seemed to have been commonplace in the day, but in the main he felt it was a waste of time and compromised his dignity, and he wouldn't do it even for princes (Jütte 2005). It was demeaning, at the bottom of it. He seems to have felt that he was being unappreciated. And you can see his point, when he writes about the case when he made the house call only to find that the gentleman of the house was at the theatre, and that the emergency wasn't really an emergency after all. It's difficult to imagine but in the 1800s the physician did not hold the prestigious place of today.

The show *Deadwood* has a great example of the working physician at a time before antibiotics were invented, dealing with the expectations of the community and not being particularly valued. Hahnemann often complained about not being paid, being paid in lottery tickets, or having to beg for his recompense.

Thus wrote Hahnemann in 1829 in a letter to the homeopath Dr Johann Heinrich Wilhelm Ehrhardt (1794-1848) in Merseburg.

Hahnemann kept to this rule even after he moved to Paris, despite the fact that his high-ranking Parisian clientèle were used to having a doctor visit them at their residence. Two years before he died, Hahnemann wrote to his friend and favourite pupil Clemens von Bönninghausen, that patients 'must come to [my] practice, if they are able to get out and about, however noble they may be'. He justifies this as follows: '[...] for I consider it to be beneath the dignity of a true doctor to have to run about after patients who are able to come to me. I will only take my carriage to visit those patients who are confined to bed.' [2] During the years he practised in Leipzig (1811-1821), it seems Hahnemann handed over all house calls to his son Friedrich [3] (Jütte 2005).

1.6.2 Virtual Consultations

It was very common for Hahnemann to treat patients by letter. This could have been a way that allowed him to maximise his time in his office with his scholarly activities. Nevertheless, it was not commonplace at the time.

The telephone has replaced the post, and many homeopaths now have call-in times for their patients to speak with them over the phone. However, a telephonic consultation generally lasts a shorter length of time than a face-to-face consultation. Markus Mortsch has shown that the ratio of personal to postal consultations in the early years of Hahnemann's Köthen practice was 3:1 (Jütte 2005).

From a legal and ethical perspective, it is important to reflect on the treatment of long-distance patients. For Hahnemann it represented no problem at all:

> And this despite the fact that many of his patients did not live in the vicinity, indeed, they often lived far away, sometimes beyond the borders of the German Empire. Nowadays, because of the extraordinary developments in transport (car, rail and plane), patients are more mobile. There are also more homeopaths than in Hahnemann's time (Jütte 2005).

1.6.3 Compliance

Treuherz and Jütte have revealed how Hahnemann's surly nature was revealed when the therapeutic relationship did not go the way he wanted it to. Of course, non-compliance puts a huge amount of strain on any relationship. And it's not as if patients were unaware of his expectations because he wrote letters to the editor many a time on the issue. Letter after letter was written to a patient exhorting them to follow his directives, be it about nutritional advice, lifestyle advice or instructions on how to take the remedy, or even about how much electricity to take.

> Esteemed Sir, You appear to believe that I have been taking other medication, or not keeping to my diet. But neither of the above

have yet come to pass. Right up to the last time I was unwell I have taken no other medication, even by olfaction, and as to my diet, I keep to it if anything excessively strictly rather than too laxly.' [5] And in a later letter this patient asks explicitly if it is really advisable to take 'the camphor tincture as prescribed' [6] for cholera prevention, as she had once before had serious side-effects from this. In this case Hahnemann bows to the patient's wishes. And on other occasions he also shows himself willing to compromise, but only in matters concerning the method of administration of homeopathic remedies (Jütte 2005).

Hahnemann had to deal with patients who decided they would break off the treatment. We know very little about his patients motives for discontinuing treatment. It is speculated that they died, that they were unhappy with their progress and went elsewhere, or that they got better and were cured. Then there was Paganini:

> And on the subject of patients who broke off their treatment, we are finally in a position to be able to solve the mystery surrounding the case-history of one of the most famous of Hahnemann's patients. It has long been a matter for speculation why the famous violinist Nicolò Paganini only consulted Hahnemann twice. It had been assumed that Hahnemann's treatment of this severely ill musician, with doses of *Pulsatilla*, had been unsuccessful. Paganini, after all, already had a long history of illness. However, as I discovered thanks to a serendipitous find in the Library of Congress in Washington D.C., the truth is actually much more banal. The doctor–patient relationship was put under severe strain due to Paganini falling madly in love with Hahnemann's young wife, Mélanie d'Hervilly, at his very first consultation. Mélanie was working at that time as her husband's assistant,

and she also treated some patients herself – though only those without means. A strongly worded letter from Mélanie to the enamoured patient, in which she gave him to understand that he could not hope for any reciprocation of his love, led to both sides preferring not to continue with the treatment (Jütte 2005).

1.6.4 Hahnemann and Money

Contemporary homeopaths are usually surprised to learn that Hahnemann asked his patients to pay up front and in cash.

We can see how his pricing and billing system worked from descriptions such as the following, which is by his pupil Dr. Franz Hartmann: 'The cheapest price for 6 numbered powders, only one of which was medicated, and either 3 or 2 of which were to be taken daily, was 16 gute Groschen. The rich were charged between 1 Thaler 8 gute Groschen and 2 Thaler – or else he had them pay the sum of 10–12 Louisd'or in advance, which after some time he demanded of them ad libitum again.' It was this last practice in particular, that of payment in advance, that some of his contemporaries felt went against the grain, despite the fact that it was common at the time for well-to-do patients to engage a personal physician on an ongoing basis, whom they paid a flat fee. This fee, however, was only payable at the end of the year, which meant the debtor could delay, reduce or even refuse payment (Jütte 2005).

His fees were by no means cheap either. Without doubt some could pay, but we know that there were complaints especially because treatment for a chronic condition with homeopathy at that time was also perceived to take longer and therefore be more expensive.

Friederike Lutze, one of Hahnemann's many female patients makes it plain in another of her letters to Hahnemann that such financial worries often added to the woes experienced by patients: '[...] my protracted illness has already cost me dearly, and the worry of how I am to meet these costs is not the least of the anxieties that weigh me down and fill me with fear.'

Ever the pragmatist, it seems that Hahnemann never took his eye off the business side of running a medical practice. He did have a lot of mouths to feed but that never stops him from being accused of putting money first.

One of the most vivid accounts we have of his views on this matter is contained in a letter he wrote to his pupil Friedrich Rummel (1793-1854), from Köthen on 19 May: '[...] and so the purely homeopathic doctor is also advised to value his infinitely better form of treatment highly enough, and thus to get a better price for it; the chronically sick, at least, should pay a monthly fee (preferably in advance), and the little man should pay an amount at each consultation and prescription – even if it is only a few Groschen each time – accipe dum dolet. In this way the doctor shall never leave empty handed, and he remains of good cheer seeing cash in return for his efforts. These small sums, if paid without fail on each and every occasion, grow imperceptibly into a larger amount, and the patient who pays each time barely notices a dent in his pocket, as he is paying only little by little, so that when he is well again, or breaks off his treatment prematurely, we are finished with him: he has nothing to demand of us, and we nothing of him. He parts from us, if not with satisfaction and thanks, then at least never with ill-will – he has forgotten all about that which he has paid out over time, and the doctor has what is reasonably due to him, and it accumulates, without any vexation on the part of the patient, in his doctor's purse.' (Jütte 2005).

1.7 Remedy versus Person in Relationship

These are the daily practicalities of running a practice, practice management. In 1810 the issues were still around money, compliance, getting clients and keeping them. 200 years later, it is not that much different. We know essentially what Hahnemann did, but we can only really guess what was going on in his mind. We can grasp the tone of some of his letters and extrapolate how he must have felt, unappreciated, neglected, undervalued. What we can never know is the degree to which he engaged with his clients, in the consultation to what extent did he manage the person as much as the case in front of him.

From the outset, the remedy, the medicine has held a place of pride and been strongly emphasised as the most crucial aspect of successful homeopathic practice. After all, homeopaths prescribe medicine, they deliver remedies to people that are suffering. They deliver help to people that have conditions and symptoms of acute and chronic diseases. Whatever your perspective, Chinese medicine, Ayurvedic medicine, homeopathic medicine, it is the intervention, the technique and the delivery of it that creates the change. Hahnemann, of course articulated so clearly the homeopathic approach to choose their medicine. And while there have been differences of opinion over the years, essentially that aspect of practice remains unchanged.

Some contemporary homeopaths have decided that they want to maximise their results and get better results so they have developed new ways and place the emphasis on different aspects of the case in order to find the best medicine possible. Scholten for one, and Sankaran for another, have developed cogent arguments, and are supported by a significant number of cures and positive results, highlighting that Hahnemann's method is not the only way to go.

1.7.1 But Where Is the Patient in All of This?

Emphasising a method to choose a drug that is going to create a cure in a patient is essentially the same as placing emphasis on the allopathic surgery or the allopathic drug. From one perspective, it makes perfect sense. After all this is what homeopathy is. Patients come, they tell their stories and their symptoms, the good doctor and homeopathic practitioner listens carefully and selects the best intervention. Patients get better.

It therefore has to be of considerable concern to all involved to realise that this is artificial and a fantasy. It also defies all reality. It also defies everything we know from modern research about a therapeutic intervention in any and all modalities of healing in any country using any system.

The relationship between the practitioner and the patient, and the practitioner's role are clearly missing in this scenario. Homeopathy is more than the pill, acupuncture is more than the needle, naturopathy is more than the anti-candida diet. We can train monkeys, and robots to do that.

The other day a patient came to see me. She had been referred from a beautician. She walked into the building looking anxious and was clearly nervous about what was in store for her. I asked her to sit down and tell me how I could assist. She burst into tears and the story came out. She is feeling terrible, has a terrible **weight** on her chest, she can't **sleep** at night. Her relationship with her husband is **disintegrating** all because of the **pressure** she constantly feels. The children have to have their homework done. She has to prepare **excellent** food. There is **pressure**. It's all down to **her**. If it doesn't happen, it is the end of the world. She cannot leave the house until the whole house is **vacuumed** and everything is tidy. She has an acute **conscience** and feels **guilty** a lot of the time. Every surface is **clean**. She cannot **relax** until everything is done and in its right place. The only thing she does to relax is **exercise** which she does at the gym four times a week for two hours in a very focused way, and she absolutely **flogs** herself and ends up **exhausted**.

Some homeopaths might hear that story and want to reach for *Arsenicum album*, and it may well be an excellent choice of remedy, or *Carcinosinum*. What I want to emphasis in this book to all homeopaths or naturopaths is that the remedy here is not the point. One of key points of this work is, when a homeopathic practitioner understands the rules of the second prescription, and how to manage a case, patients get better, when they understand what is a new symptom, a return of an old symptom, when they understand what an aggravation is, patients have better outcomes.

Furthermore, the homeopath that engages with a client as I did with this woman, is going to get better results, and have a more thriving practice than the brilliant homeopath that prescribes the similar medicine at the outset.

I sat with her 10 minutes not writing or asking or really doing anything while she cried and cried. I didn't even really reach for the tissues. And I certainly didn't attempt to rescue her or make it any better. I just sat there and *was with* her. After a while she looked at me and said I never said this to anyone before.

'This all started when this terrible thing happened to my sister'.

I wondered what it was and wondered if she died, if she'd been killed in a car crash or something.

'My sister's husband cheated on her and everybody in the suburb knows about it, and it has been a really hard time for me over the last two years.'

I was surprised by this response because I was anticipating something different. Of course knowing that I should not really be anticipating anything at all. Nevertheless I thought it would be a different answer than it was. I asked why it affected her so much. She said,

'I've never told anyone this but I was completely in love with him when I was younger, we had a relationship and eventually we split up and he ended up marrying my sister.'

She burst into tears again. She hadn't told her best friend who was her sister, nor anyone else in the family. Now I can't tell you if the medicine which I've given her has helped. I've no idea to what degree she can get better because I haven't seen her yet for a second time. What I do know is that she has had a therapeutic intervention which has made a difference for her, and with the combination of a homeopathic remedy, and the experience of being listened to, a difference has been made in her life. This is the point of this book. Being a homeopath is not about the remedy. The remedy is certainly a large part of a process, and an important part, and the more accurate the selection of the remedy the better, but it is not the full story. This mistaken over emphasis on the right remedy has done homeopathy a massive disservice over the years.

From start to finish, homeopaths that know how to manage the case, manage people, and manage themselves, are more effective homeopaths than technicians that have their noses glued to the computer learning everything there is to know about the keynotes of some obscure small medicine. It is not my intention to be overly controversial by saying these things, rather to point out that a balance needs to be restored in our thinking, teaching, and practice of homeopathic medicine. There is a disclaimer though: I am absolutely not saying, nor believe, that a homeopath needs to be a therapist. I do not believe this is the case and I don't believe that a homeopath needs to be a counselor nor have a substantial amount of training and psychotherapy or counseling. They need foundations and fundamentals.

Arguing this case is not to be lazy either. I am not saying any old polychrest will do because of course this is not the case either. We have a duty to get as close as we can with homeopathy to assist our patients and clients.

This is what I mean by remedy versus person. There's a strange amount of emphasis in homeopathy on the goal. 'He's a Scholten prescriber or she is a Bönninghausen prescriber'. To my mind, this is equivalent to looking into a field of sheep and being told that they're different in some way. I can't really tell the difference myself sometimes. There are different styles of homeopathy and the distinction between them is different. It's not so much about method but approach. What I mean by approach is a traditional one in which the interaction looks something like this: 'I am the homeopath, and you are the patient. I will make you better if you take this remedy.'

As I argued in my *Case Taking* book in 2010, this approach was superseded by many homeopaths in the 1970s and 80s after the influence of post-Jungian thought, and the adoption of many of the attitudes and postures that he developed. Homeopaths started to take cases and see patients in a different way, and started to ask different questions, and as a consequence give different and sometimes better remedies.

As my friend and colleague Brian Kaplan has pointed out in his lectures and 2001 book, more than any other, the difference between homeopaths is whether they are there in the room fully and consciously with a patient using an approach that could be best be described as psychodynamic or person centred. A doctor being a doctor with a white coat is often a very useful thing. A doctor being a doctor who is completely present in the moment with a patient is an even better thing. It's exactly the same with osteopathy and midwifery. It is not about being a therapist or a counselor; it is about being there fully and consciously.

1.8 Other Literature

In 2008, a book, *Principles and Practice of Homoeopathic Case Management* was published by Nigam. The first part of this book examines various historical interpretations of what makes up a human being. There is a section devoted to concepts of disease and remedy before 20 pages on case management towards the end of the book, much from Ian Watson's *Guide to the Methodologies of Homeopathy*. In addition, there are excellent chapters on case management to be found in the works of Close, Roberts, Kent, Sankaran, Little and Koehler. Substantial portions of them are reproduced here. In addition, the work of de Schepper (2004) in *Achieving and Maintaining the Simillimum* is excellent and a must read.

1.9 Conclusion

The busy and thriving contemporary homeopath is able to grasp the dual pillars of case management. These pillars include both traditional case management from the masters, and modern principles of case management. The latter comprises complex case management that come from working at the coalface with patients from all fields of life, living lifestyles of which Hahnemann could not have dreamed.

Part Two

Getting Busy | Traditional Case Management Strategies, Principles and Techniques

In this section you will:
1. Become familiar with the authors who have contributed to the traditional literature
2. Identify the history, theory, and philosophy around the second prescription
3. Learn the opinions of homeopathic leaders, Little, Vithoulkas, Kent, De Schepper
4. Gain insight into when to repeat the remedy and when to change it

Part Two

Getting Busy | Traditional Case Management Strategies, Principles and Techniques

Part Two | Contents

Chapter 2 | Foundations
    2.1 Introduction
    2.2 Follow-up Case Taking
    2.3 Structure and Bedrock
    2.4 The Basics | Hahnemann's Classification of Disease
    2.5 What is an Aggravation?
    2.6 What is a Proving Symptom?
    2.7 What is a Return of an Old Symptom?
    2.8 What is a New Symptom?

Chapter 3 | History
    3.1 Evaluation of the Patient's Response
    3.2 History of the editions of the *Organon*

Chapter 4 | Principles
4.1 The Second Prescription
    4.1.1 Hahnemann
    4.1.2 Roberts
    4.1.3 Chatterjee
    4.1.4 Kent: The Second Prescription
    4.1.5 Kent: What the People Should Know

Chapter 5 | Observe, Understand and Act
5.1 Remedy Reactions
    5.1.1 Hahnemannn
    5.1.2 Roberts
    5.1.3 Kent: Prognosis after Observing the Action of the Remedy

Chapter 6 | Specific Techniques
6.1 When This Happens...Do That
    6.1.1 Sherr
        Nothing happens | No change
        The Total Positive Reaction
        The Total Negative Reaction
        The Partially Positive and Negative Reaction
    6.1.2 Vithoulkas
        Disadvantages of the Graphs
    6.1.3 Henriques
    6.1.4 De Schepper
    6.1.5 Summary and Collective Wisdom

Chapter 7 | Repetition of the Dose
7.1 4th edition of the *Organon* - Opinions
    7.1.1 Hussey
    7.1.2 Close

7.1.3 Banerjee: The First Prescription
7.1.4 Banerjee: The Second Prescription
7.1.5 Close Again

Chapter 8 | The Rich Landscape of Posology
8.1 Hahnemann's Timeline in the Development and use of the 50 Millesimal Potencies
8.2 Critical Thinking

Chapter 9 | Best Practice, Potency and Administration
9.1 The Luck of the Draw
9.2 Burnett on Potency
9.3 Kent's Flexibility and the Endless Field
9.4 Hahnemann's Flexibility
9.5 Little's Best Practice
9.6 Lippe

Part Two

Getting Busy | Traditional Case Management Strategies, Principles and Techniques

The first prescription is not the most difficult. The second one is the most difficult. We see a new picture coming and prescribe on it too soon. That is the most common mistake. We need to wait to make the second prescription, and not spoil the very good first prescription. If you spoil a case in this way, go back to the first prescription and see from there where you went wrong. It is usually in the second prescription that you will find your error. Heudens-Mast (1998)

Chapter Two | Foundations

In this chapter you will:

1. Learn the underpinnings and theory of the second prescription
2. Grasp the fundamental concepts that relate to this part of the process
3. Explore Hahnemann's classification of disease

Chapter 2

Foundations

2.1 Introduction

The title of this second section of this book is *Getting Busy | Traditional Case Management Strategies, Principles and Techniques*. I am convinced that thriving homeopathic practice can only be partially attributed to accurate medicine selection, and has as much if not more to do with how to manage people and apply management principles. This part is a one-stop shop of who has said what. Furthermore, it provides rationale for why they have said it. As emphasised previously, knowing when to intervene, knowing exactly what the remedy that you gave three weeks ago has done, and being able to identify exactly what needs to be done next provides more value to a patient and one's own practice. These key points are crucial to know.

Homeopaths and students alike often look at their professional environment and ask questions. Why am I not busier? One of the many reasons is that the skills of the second prescription are not well taught, integrated or emphasised in their training. There are a number of reasons why. The focus is erroneously often on the first prescription. Moreover, it's hard to teach and it's often not interesting. Teaching the skills of evaluating the patient's response requires endless practice to integrate confidently. It also implies a case must be fully understood in an individual training session, which includes, the first consultation, and the reasons for the prescription. Only then, you can get onto the point of the session, which is to understand what happened when the first medicine was given, and how to decipher the results appropriately. It's a long session. Graduates are often left to work it out themselves at the coalface in their own clinics, with real patients and by themselves. And given its importance in clinic maintenance and getting great results, this approach is perilous. One of the problems with emphasising this aspect of homeopathy is that it's not very sexy. Just ask anyone who runs a homeopathic college, or course, or a postgraduate programme. They will tell you the same thing. People don't want to hear about Bönninghausen's 10 strategies of case management, or Kent's 12 remedy reactions, or Vithoulkas' 22 ways to deal with a remedy reaction. They'd much rather hear about the latest sea creature proving. It's not riveting stuff by any stretch of the imagination, and in my experience of running postgraduate programmes, participants often choose that moment to have a snooze when you say the words, 'right let's revise what we know about remedy reactions'.

In fact it's just like tennis. Years ago, in my twenties, I had the good fortune to be a tennis groupie in Europe one summer. For months, I followed some friends and other tennis players around on the circuit, in the south of France helping out where I could, doing the shopping, doing the washing and trying to look fabulous. While I didn't succeed in the glamour department, I certainly did succeed in watching a lot of tennis.

And here's what I learned. Tennis players are weird, even professional ones like the friends with whom I was travelling. When tennis players get on a court to practice, they stand there and they hit the ball to each other. They do this for ages. Even though this bears no reality whatsoever to exactly what goes on in a tennis match. What happens in a tennis match is exactly the opposite. Most of the tennis match involves serving the ball and receiving the ball. Except on clay and on artificial surfaces, there is very little in the way of rallies in any form of tennis anywhere in the world. And yet even with this knowledge, tennis players still warm up by hitting the ball to each other to practice. It's crazy.

It's the same thing in homeopathy. Homeopaths study homeopathy and practice homeopathy as if the only thing that happens in homeopathy is finding the right remedy the first time. It's not real. What happens most in homeopathy is long rallies, exactly the opposite of tennis, and this is what homeopaths should practice. Homeopaths should in fact be practising their second prescription skills four times more often than they practice their searching for the right remedy skills because this is what they do four times as much or more than any other thing in the work of being a homeopath.

The skills of the second prescription are what homeopaths do most of the time in the 21st century. These skills include evaluating one-sided cases, working with non-compliant patients, addressing dependency issues with drugs and alcohol, and raising awareness of lifestyle issues. Now this focus may have been different in Hahnemann's time because in those days for him, and in some parts of the world such as India still, this is what practitioners mainly do. But for the rest of us in the western world especially, in New Zealand and Australia, in North America, the UK, and in Europe, homeopaths are still wrestling with these realities:

- Patients do what they want and they have their own set of rules.
- Homeopathy at the coalface bears little resemblance to how it was described in a textbook that was written in 1900, or to the *Organon* written in 1810.

To thrive in homeopathic practice, the issues talked about in this chapter far outweigh the importance of learning the keynotes of yet other remedy that you can look up or look for in any textbook. The indications of *Causticum* are in the books. Don't worry about it. They're not going anywhere and they're likely not going to change much. But having to manage a patient with diabetes who has come to you to help them give up smoking, and who has a tightness in the chest and low energy levels, with anxiety and going through a divorce is going to require skilful management, and it is these skills that are far more important.

The purpose of this part of the book is therefore to assist homeopaths in achieving better clinical outcomes. In addition, it is a guide to assist practitioners in keeping their patients, making fewer mistakes, and developing better skills to prescribe the second prescription. As homeopathic practitioners, we see a new picture coming and prescribe on it too soon. That is the most common mistake. We need to wait to make the second prescription. Ultimately, the objective is to provide clarity around what is meant by *The Second Prescription*. The second prescription is quite simply the prescription given after the one that worked.

2.2 Follow-up Case Taking

A word needs to be said about case taking in the subsequent consultations to the first. Follow-up case taking is significantly different from the skills and activities in the first consultation. The intention is different. In the first consultation, the intention is to get as much information about the characteristic symptoms of the disease, or the whole person to make an accurate prescription. In the follow-up consultation, the intention is to determine how far along the patient has come. The skills required are different. What has happened since the patient took the prescribed remedy? The answer to this question is crucial. And after having established what's happened, you can then act and make decisions to move forward.

I often find myself beginning the second consultation with something like, 'it's been forever, how long is it exactly since we last met?' Obviously I know, but I want to know what they say. What they say is very interesting. It gives them the opportunity now to tell the story of what has happened in the interim. Of course, in this situation the best thing is to remain silent and just take notes so you can see if the symptoms have changed, the condition has changed, or of the patient has changed in some way.

With eczema, with pain, with a migraine, it's easy to determine what is going on. In the first consultation, the homeopath will have determined exactly the symptom picture, and drawn a line in the sand. The work of a follow-up consultation is to simply measure how far the patient has come from that place. But it is much more difficult and much harder to measure something like menstrual pain or hayfever or anxiety or depression because of the cyclical nature of the symptoms and because it requires both subjective and objective observation.

Determining if symptoms in a case have improved is one thing, and determining if the focus of the case has shifted is another. Have the sufferings moved from something deeper, more internal, more serious to something more superficial more external and less intense? Ultimately, answering this question is the goal. Symptoms either go away completely, or come less often and with less intensity. Observation skills are fundamental, and looking at all the details is crucial. With questioning skills, there is really very little difference between the first and second and the tenth consultation. A physical examination may be necessary, and again the skills are usually the same between the first and the twentieth consultation.

When it comes to recording symptoms though, there may be a difference. Going back carefully through the first consultation is important to identify any symptoms that may show improvement. And of course, the patient may not remember or very often not attribute any change to something else. This is just a simple annoying but real consequence of the fact that when patients change, their capacity to observe also changes and they may not attribute accurately the reason for any particular changes.

New information constantly comes up in subsequent follow-up consultations. It's important to clearly identify any new information in the case notes because this information needs to be added to the original material. It may be stories from the childhood, or it may be further characteristic symptoms that were not articulated at first consultation.

For the most part, it is the same questioning technique that is used as in the first consultation, keeping silent, tracing the picture of the disease, acting as if you don't quite understand, allowing the patient to tell the story (Gray 2010). In addition, check carefully that the patient took the medicine as directed, and if not why not? At the end of the day, it's a methodical process of going through the original notes from the first consultation, and clarifying what has gone on, to what extent there has been change, and to what extent is that change heading in a positive direction. Ultimately, we are looking for a clear remedy response.

Posture

- 'How are things with you?'

Reflective Questions

- What was the reaction to the first medicine prescribed?
- What are our expectations?
- What is the prognosis?
- Is there a more suitable medicine?
- Is there a more suitable potency?
- Is there a more suitable repetition program?
- Are there any obstacles that prevent or hinder recovery?
- Is referral for medical testing or other professional treatment or advice necessary?
- What is the medicine response?
- What are the various responses that could take place?
- What do the various possible responses indicate?

So overall, the principles of the follow-up consultation are similar to the initial consultation, but the intention is different. What has happened?

- Changes in lifestyle/circumstances since the last interview
- Maintaining causes
- Category of case - simple, chronic, complicated
- Remedy storage and administration compliance
- Additional stresses
- Adjunct therapies / medications
- Memory of condition?
- Hering's direction

All this makes the next part more simple, 'What will I do now?'

In terms of recording the consultation, best practice determines that there should be clear file organisation, if written notes, kept in a locked filing cabinet. Storage of previous information must be in an easy-to-gain-access format and this is mandatory. If notes are electronically taken or in a patient management system they need to be backed up and safe. In addition, notes need to have a cover sheet, the remedy name, date etc (Weir 2003). Direct speech, abbreviations need to be kept to a minimum and translatable, the weighting given and individual symptoms with underlining, numbering, highlighting should also be transparent. Notes on all interim correspondence and suggestions, from texts and emails should be included.

2.3 Structure and Bedrock

Evaluating the action of a remedy is possible when you know exactly the starting point. Many homeopaths forget that Hahnemann gives us our road map of where we're going when it comes to evaluating the patients response in the *Organon of Medicine*, the ultimate do-it-yourself manual.

2.4 The Basics | Hahnemann's Classification of Disease

Although reading the *Organon* can be laborious, and it may seem outdated at times, it remains a valuable representation of the history and thinking of Hahnemann. The *Organon* is a book of ideals, of homeopathic philosophy and practical applications with directives and warnings.

The Origins of the First Edition

1796. Published article in Hufeland's *Medical Journal*, An Essay on a New Principle for Ascertaining the Curative Powers of Drugs.
1805. *Medicine of Experience*
1810. *Organon of the Rational Art of Healing.* The first edition was not translated until 1913 by Charles Wheeler (JM Dent - Everyman edition).

The Six Editions

1st published in Leipzig Germany 1810
The translations are important. The 4th edition was published in 1829 and translated into English in Dublin in 1833 and Pennsylvania 1836. The 5th edition 1833, translated by Dudgeon in London in 1849 by which time the 4th edition had been reprinted several times so both editions circulated on both sides of the Atlantic leading to different interpretations of potency selection and posology. The same phenomenon occurred with French and Spanish translations.
5th edition published in Germany 1833
6th edition completed in 1842 *"the most nearly perfected of all"* he wrote to his publishers.

The Evolution, Changes, Alterations and Improvements

Most important changes are those of Aphorisms 269-272 regarding potency & dosage in *chronic diseases*.
Various attempts were made to get Hahnemann's second wife Melanie to release the 6th edition. The incredibly high price tag thwarted each attempt.
1921. The 6th edition was finally available for translation and publication.

Layout

Translator's Preface
Introduction to various editions
Contents
Introduction to the work
294 Aphorisms (§)
Footnotes and Appendix

In specific aphorisms in the *Organon*, Hahnemann lays out and articulates his classification of disease. While he crafted the book in paragraph form, it is sometimes a lot easier to conceptualise when perceived as a model.

Foundations

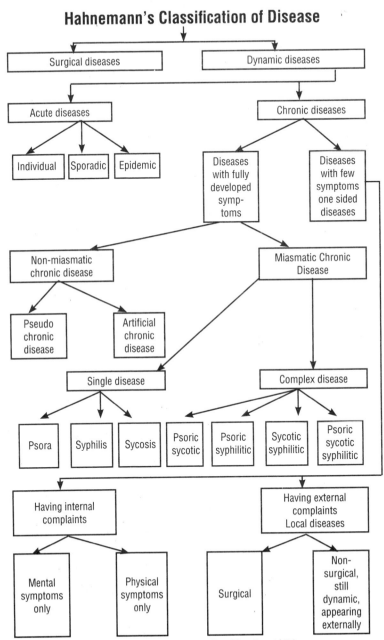

Figure One | Hahnemann's Classification of Disease.
Adapted from Hahnemann (2005) and Asok Kumar Das (1998).

Furthermore, it is good to be reminded of the true context of homeopathic prescribing. If the condition is a minor indisposition, work with the diet.

Aphorism 150 If a patient complains of one or more trivial symptoms, that have been only observed a short time previously, the physician should not regard this as a fully developed disease that requires serious medical aid. A slight alteration in the diet and regimen will usually suffice to dispel such an indisposition.

Aphorism 151 But if the patient complains of a few violent sufferings, the physician will usually find, on investigation, several other symptoms besides, although of a slighter character, which furnish a complete picture of the disease.

Aphorism 152 The worse the acute disease is, of so much the more numerous and striking symptoms is it generally composed, but with so much the more certainty may a suitable remedy for it be found, if there be a sufficient number of medicines known, with respect to their positive action, to choose from. Among the lists of symptoms of many medicines it will not be difficult to find one from whose separate disease elements an antitype of curative artificial disease, very like the totality of the symptoms of the natural disease, may be constructed, and such a medicine is the desired remedy.

Aphorism 153 In this search for a homoeopathic specific remedy, that is to say, in this comparison of the collective symptoms of the natural disease with the list of symptoms of known medicines, in order to find among these an artificial morbific agent corresponding by similarity to the disease to be cured, the *more striking, singular, uncommon and peculiar* (characteristic) signs and symptoms of the case of disease are chiefly and most solely to be kept in view; for it is *more particularly these that very similar ones in the* *list of symptoms of the selected medicine must correspond to*, in order to constitute it most suitable for effecting the cure. The more general and undefined symptoms: loss of appetite, headache, debility, restless sleep, discomfort, and so forth, demand but little attention when of that vague and indefinite character, if they cannot be more accurately described, as symptoms of such a general nature are observed in almost every disease and from almost every drug (Hahnemann 1921).

As well as the structure, it is important to remember the absolute basics. So many students and practitioners get confused by misidentifying the reaction to the remedy.

2.5 What is an Aggravation?

An aggravation is nothing other than a magnification of the symptoms that were there previously. It's as simple as that.

Most of the available literature agrees that, if after using a centesimal potency, an aggravation occurs, the remedy is generally stopped and a period of waiting occurs. This is slightly different to the instructions in the sixth edition of the *Organon* where an aggravation, which generally happens towards the end of treatment, necessitates a period of waiting and observing. Again in the situation, the rule is to wait.

Kent, Vithoulkas and various other writers in the Kentian tradition consider aggravation as a good thing. There are many textbooks that go into significant depth about a true and false aggravation. Assuming that the remedy has been a partial similar, if an aggravation occurs, it is usually argued that this is a positive step. It is an indication that the vital force of the patient has been stimulated, has reacted against and pushed against the action of the remedy, and the magnification of the symptoms are a sure sign that improvement is on the way. In diagrammatical form, this spike in the pre-existing symptoms at the beginning of treatment indicates a positive reaction even though there might be some discomfort involved. It is the duration of this discomfort that is the issue. Discomfort is miserable. Pain is unpleasant. And so when the patient rings in the middle of an aggravation and says, 'this is happening', and the homeopath indicates that this is a good sign, this news can be met with some bemusement on behalf the patient.

This is the art of case management at its heart. Managing a patient through an aggravation without alarming the patient, allowing the remedy to do its job and for the patient to come back to a restful place is a difficult task of management. So often it is not clear exactly what is going on. A week later or a month later, it's very easy to see what has happened. But in the middle of that crisis or aggravation, it is sometimes not clear. Here is the point where many homeopaths have acted inappropriately and antidoted remedies, or moved on to a new remedy and not allowed the action of the remedy to run its course.

Although premature selection of another remedy is to be avoided at all costs, it's difficult to put into practice. The patient is anxious and in pain and asking questions. The homeopath tries to do the right thing. To do it well, there must be clarity that this is in fact the true aggravation. Then and only then can the patient truly trust the homeopath.

The only correct course of action during an aggravation is to wait. If there's anything new that comes along, then it is not an aggravation and another course of action is necessary. If it's a return of an old symptom, or a proving symptom, then it is not an aggravation.

2.6 What is a Proving Symptom?

It might be difficult in the moment to perceive the difference between a proving symptom and an aggravation. However, if the experience of the patient is in fact a proving of the remedy, then this is significantly different to an aggravation. Careful questioning and a sound, grounded disposition is very important in this situation. An aggravation is described as a magnification of what was there before. A proving on the other hand is obviously a symptom or series of symptoms that can be attributed to the remedy that has been taken. The only way to determine this is by having access to the proving documents of the remedy that's been given.

These are clearly identified in Hahnemann's *Materia Medica Pura*, *Chronic Diseases* or Allen's *Encyclopedia*. These primary source books are absolute necessities in clinical practice. When it comes to more modern provings, only access to the proving data through the web, professional software, or published proving monographs will ensure that the homeopath can be clear that what is happening for the patient is the development of a proving symptom.

By stopping and waiting, usually after short amount of time, the symptoms start diminishing, the intensity of the symptoms lessen, and the patient returns to the same place before taking the remedy or better. Either way, it is crucial to determine if this is a genuine proving or an aggravation.

2.7 What is a Return of an Old Symptom?

The return of an old symptom is when the patient begins to develop symptoms from previous points in the patient's life after having taken a homeopathic remedy. The return of old symptoms are almost always a good sign. It is important that this information is relayed and articulated clearly to the patient to mitigate anxiety and reduce the chances of having the patient interfere or intervene inappropriately in the treatment plan.

In my experience, the return of old symptoms can include anything, including physical symptoms such as skin problems or headaches, those that last occurred in childhood, and even revisiting emotional hurt, pain and trauma that happened in the past.

At the end of the day, it's about intensity and just how long the patient can sustain uncomfortable symptoms. It may be a completely new concept to clients to learn that they need to go through a period of time, hopefully a short amount of time, where they need to experience symptoms that they had before. Like aggravations, and proving symptoms, the return of old symptoms necessitate the stopping of any homeopathic remedy. Only in some cases that are pretty rare will any continuation through the symptoms be required. Thus in all situations so far, we stop the remedy and observe. How long we observe, what happens during the time of observation and how this is articulated to the client is very important. The client needs and deserves legitimate answers to the questions about why this is happening and how long will it take. 'How long shall I wait?' 'Can I trust you?'

2.8   What is a New Symptom?

Anything new that happens after administering a remedy also requires the patient to stop taking the medicine, and for the practitioner to observe and wait. Jeremy Sherr teaches, 'the simillimum does nothing new.' This implies that if new symptoms appear, then the remedy that has been given can only be a partial similar. There is nothing wrong in prescribing partial similars. In the hands of confident practitioners who know what they are doing, this approach is a good and legitimate way to get to resolve symptoms.

Chapter Three | History

In this chapter you will:

1. Learn the historical context and precedents
2. Identify the authors that have articulated the basics
3. Understand the fundamentals of the landscape of traditional case management

Chapter 3
History

3.1 Evaluation of the Patient's Response

With this foundation established, understanding Hahnemann's classification, understanding the immediate difference between an aggravation, a return of an old symptom, a new symptom and a proving symptom, it is possible to proceed and explore in more depth just what to do when the patient returns.

Many homeopaths forget to use the words,

- *measure*
- *outcome*
- *result*
- *strategy*
- *solution*

in their follow-up consultations. Some perceive these words as overly allopathic, and argue that conventional words and concepts do not reflect the tone of homeopathy and complementary medicine. To my mind, these are fundamental words to use in follow-up consultations. They engage clients. They assist in focusing our minds and our patients' minds on just how far they have come or not in the intervening time since we last saw them. This evaluation stage is really important to get right and master. Jon Gamble (2005) in his introduction argued that this is an excellent way to practice. That is, at the beginning of a course of treatment, especially in a case with few characteristics, apply a statistically significant therapeutic medicine, based on traditional use and evidence, and then manage the case accurately and clearly as a larger totality prescription emerges from the continuing consultations.

Some cases

A man came to see me with digestive troubles. I've shown this case numerous times on video to audiences and students. Everyone is entertained because in the course of telling me his symptoms, this man gets into the most extraordinary positions and makes incredible gestures that make him look like, amongst other things, a monkey. He tells me about his problems. His energy levels slump, he asks me why I think that despite eating so much food he never puts on any weight, he shows me his chest and says, 'look at this, it's so narrow, where does all the food go'? and then proceeds to give me an incredible description of the tubercular miasmatic disease, in all of its forms. Clearly this man needs *Tuberculinum bov*, *Phosphorus*, or *Iodium*. On returning, he sat down in the chair and looked across and said, 'thank you very much, I am 135% better. I've measured it and I am 135% better. Thank you very much.' Now this does not happen that often where patients are able to articulate in some way, or even accurately describe just how much better they are with their presenting symptom or how they are in themselves. This case is very different to another patient that I had.

History

An older gentleman came to see me in about 1996. He was very large, obese in fact, and had a thick central European accent. The story was quite extraordinary. He had recently been hit by a car and had to go to hospital. He took some medications but couldn't really explain to me what they were because English was his second language and he didn't bring the medications with him on his visit. It sounded like he was on blood pressure medication, thyroid medication and something else. He talked about not being able to sleep at night, and he talked about resisting going to the hospital when the ambulance came to pick him up after he'd been hit by the car. I asked him why he had resisted going to the hospital when he was so hurt. He didn't want to tell me. But eventually he said that the last time he was in hospital was 1942. He told me this extraordinary story about how during the war he was experimented on in a concentration camp hospital and given injections. He remembers rats and he remembers the rats running through the sleeping boys in the concentration camp and feeling terrible after the injections that he received on a regular basis. He describes himself as *half dead*. He remembers the rats from the hospital and the rats trying to eat the boys. He remembered feeling dreamy and he remembered floating. He also remembered being rescued by a Gestapo officer who smuggled him out of the camp. He was eventually rescued and found by his father in 1946.

If that wasn't enough, he found himself a refugee in Australia in 1968 after the Russian invasion of Czechoslovakia. These days he made souvenirs and cobbled together his life. He said that he didn't have many friends. He spent time making souvenirs for the tourists. There are a number of other aspects of the case but essentially that was it. The result of the injections was that he had never been able to sustain an erection and had never had a relationship. He was numb 'down there'. The remedy chosen for him was *Opium*.

He came back after four weeks. The response was extraordinary. He talked about a cleaning sensation in his chest and in the stomach, and not needing to take the conventional medicine any more. He thanked me. He asked for another bottle of the homeopathic remedy (he ignored my instructions to just take three doses of *Opium* 1M and had taken the whole bottle). He was better in himself and he was better with the symptoms, his energy levels had improved.

These examples serve to remind us that measuring change is sometimes very difficult.

3.2 History of the Editions of the *Organon*

It is a feature of our profession that whoever was the teacher affects the student so much; it really matters. There are some astonishing teachers of homeopathy and some shockers as well. There is an over reliance across the board in the landscape of homeopathic education on personality, charisma as opposed to accuracy and curriculum. Unfortunately when it comes to a significant amount of homeopathic education, the personal opinion and experience of an individual trainer may create another emphasis or a lack of balance on the perspectives of students. When it comes to case management, it absolutely depends on who taught you. The perspectives, cultural angles, reading or lack of reading of the teacher utterly impacts the student's understanding. Crucially it depends on the edition of the *Organon* from which the teacher is teaching.

The very basic question is: Did your teacher teach you the fourth, fifth or sixth edition of the *Organon of Medicine?* Some people may have been taught all of the above. The student's understanding about case management will be fundamentally pinned to this point. Understanding this will enable you to grasp why your teachers said what they said and why they perhaps differ.

Educated in history before turning to homeopathic medicine, my understanding of history is that it has very little of anything to do with the past. History has everything to do with the present. It is only through understanding where we come from, and the landscape of different issues that we can fully appreciate where we are currently. History is nothing more than answering the question, 'how did we get here?' It is asking and then answering the question, 'what on earth happened that got us to this place?' When it comes to understanding traditional case management in homeopathy it is no different. Along with de Schepper (2004), Little's historical grasp on the crucial differences in the 4th, 5th and 6th editions of the *Organon* of Medicine in *Hahnemann's Advanced Methods Part 1: Hahnemannian Homeopathy,* make his discourse on case management mandatory reading.

In this excellent article he explores the transformation that Hahnemann went through publishing different versions of the *Chronic Disease,* the fifth in 1839 and the fifth and sixth editions of the *Organon* 1833 and 1842. His ideas changed over time. But early on he argued that as long as there was progressive improvement, all repetition of any dose of any medicine was forbidden. This fourth edition approach, the single-dose wait and watch method was adopted and used by his colleagues and generations ever since. But even as early as the 1820s he was wanting to improve this method especially because of resistant chronic diseases. In 1833 in the fifth edition of the *Organon* and the third, fourth and fifth editions of *The Chronic Diseases,* he clearly argued that the liquid solution was superior to dry pellets. He also argued for succussion of the remedy before administration, arguing the repeated doses were by now permissible. Prescribing in this way allowed for adjusting of the dose to suit the individual patient. The remedy could be succussed any number of times just before ingestion depending on the sensitivity of the client. These are the views of the fifth edition of the *Organon*. Still later he changed is mind again. It is important to read Little's article and de Schepper's book to understand how his thinking shifted throughout this period to the extent that he was comfortable with prescribing as long as there was steady improvement. The dose could be repeated depending on the nature of the remedy, the constitution, and the disease (Little 1996-2007).

As a complement to Little's clarity, all students and practitioners should read and re-read de Schepper's (2004) *Achieving and Maintaining the Similimum*, chapters 3-5.

Chapter Four | Principles

In this chapter you will:

1. Identify Hahnemann's directives
2. Critically think about these principles for the homeopath in current times
3. Understand the different approaches of other authors and commentators

Chapter 4

Principles

4.1 The Second Prescription

4.1.1 Hahnemann

In the literature, there is plenty of advice to guide the second prescriptions. Keep impeccable records, avoid haste, and cultivate the art of waiting. These skills and demonstrations of artfulness underpin busy practice.

Aphorism 2: "The highest ideal of cure is the rapid, gentle and permanent restoration of health;"

Aphorism 154: "if the disease is not very long standing it will generally be removed or extinguished by the first dose of the simillimum without considerable disturbance"

Aphorism 156: "if the potency is too low (crude), especially in sensitive patients, it will commonly cause a disturbance for it is impossible for the medicine and the disease to cover one another as exactly as two triangles. This slight disturbance is easily done away with by the vital force"

Aphorism 158: "a slight Homoeopathic aggravation in the first few hours is very good portent that the acute disease will yield to the first dose. This is as it should be as the medicinal disease must be stronger than the malady to overpower it" (Hahnemann 1921).

This is sound advice. It is easy to follow and replicate.

4.1.2 Roberts

Roberts also outlines the issues.

> After studying a chronic case and after deciding on the remedy, having given each symptom its proper evaluation, and having administered the simillimum, we expect some action, some response. After the patient shows the desired reaction, there may and probably will come a time when the physician is called upon to meet a symptom picture once more. This is the time when he must consider the second prescription.
>
> Strictly speaking, the first prescription is the prescription that first reacts.
>
> A physician may make a mistake and not select a remedy that is similar, consequently with no reaction. Thus while we may seem to be looking for a second prescription, we are in reality looking for a first prescription to which the patient will react. In other words, the prescription must be considered as the simillimum. Unless the patient reacts to the administration of a remedy and it has produced an effect, it is not a true prescription, for it is quite evident that it is not the simillimum. It is really bungling.
>
> The second prescription may be a repetition of the first.
>
> On the other hand, the reaction may have been such that an antidote is required; or the first remedy having taken care of a

part of the symptoms, a complement of the first prescription may be demanded.

In order to meet the situation intelligently, after the remedy has reacted, the case must be thoroughly restudied.

In general, if the first prescription has had a beneficial reaction, that remedy should be allowed to complete its work to the fullest extent. In such conditions, the second prescription would be a repetition of the first; and since a remedy should not be changed without very good reasons, it is probable that the remedy may be repeated at the necessary intervals through a whole range of potencies, securing the full amount of good from each potency before passing on to the next.

The reaction to the correct prescription is that the striking features, the peculiar features, the concomitant symptoms on which the choice of the remedy was based, are the first symptoms to be removed; thus the guiding symptoms of the case have been obliterated. The picture has been almost erased, and only the trivial symptoms are left. Now if the remedy is repeated at this stage, the cycle of cure is broken; for the guiding symptoms will surely return only when the action of the remedy is exhausted. If there is no interference with the action of the remedy, the indications which give us the clue to our next step will present themselves. One of the hardest things for a physician to do is to keep his hands off at this stage. If the remedy is administered at this stage we will find an intermingling of drug symptoms, so that no intelligent prescription can be made.

If the first prescription has not acted curatively, or it has not been permitted to act to its fullest extent, it is impossible to get second observations; but suppose that the first prescription was correct, and that it has been given plenty of time to act without interference:

If the case has come to a standstill or if the first prescription has caused changes in the symptomatology that remain, that do not vary greatly for some little time, it is time to go over the case again with the second prescription in mind. While these changes are going on, no orderly symptoms can be gathered and no rational observations made. If we have given time for the proper reaction and the fuller development of the case, having allowed the natural period of rest, the time has come to make a minute observation upon the return of the original symptoms, which should be our first consideration.

They may not return as strong or marked as they appeared before the first prescription, but we must look carefully for the return of the original symptoms. It is while the action of the remedy is going on that the vital principle is re-established in the economy; and while this process is going on we will not find the return of the original symptoms. The length of time varies in different individuals and in different remedies; it may be a few weeks and it may be months.

Now what are we to do at this time? Without symptoms we cannot prescribe intelligently. Symptoms are the only guide to the remedy. The duty of the physician is plainly marked: to await the return of the symptom picture. In chronic conditions we may be quite sure that the symptoms will return, for it is very rarely that we can cure a case with one prescription. When the symptoms return, they may be changed as to their intensity; sometimes they return in a less intense form and sometimes they are increased in intensity. The fact that the original symptoms return is a very good omen. It shows that the first prescription was correct. In this case there is very little that we need in the way of information beyond this, because we know that the remedy was right and the patient can be cured. In this case the remedy must be a repetition of the first prescription.

Another class of cases we must consider are those that present a number of new symptoms which appear to take the place of the old symptoms. The old symptoms do not return, but are replaced by an entirely different symptom group. In these conditions we must restudy the case entirely in the pathogenesis of the remedy we have already given, and find if the new symptoms that have appeared are in the pathogenesis of the remedy. If this is so, we may find that this condition comes from a partial proving of the remedy, or we may find that these appear from a different cause. This is an important point. We must determine from the patient whether he has ever had any of these symptoms before in any former sicknesses or under any other conditions. We must go over these points carefully to see if we cannot elicit from the patient the history of these symptoms. Sometimes we get these relationships from the patient and sometimes from the family.

If these are old symptoms, we not only chose our first prescription correctly but it has eliminated the newest symptoms and uncovered an older layer, in the proper order of cure; but if we can get no history of the patient having had these symptoms before, and if they are not in the pathogenesis of the remedy, we have made a mistake in the first prescription, and it has changed the direction of the disease. Here, if it is possible, we must antidote the remedy.

After having given the antidotal remedy and a little time for the patient to rest, we should study the case again from the beginning; and the second remedy should correspond more particularly to the new symptoms than to the old, but both the present symptoms and the former symptoms must be considered. If we do our work carefully, this second prescription will cause the new symptoms to disappear and it will probably remove the old symptoms as well.

We may have to repeat the process several times before we really overcome the difficulty, but each time that it is done makes the next step more difficult and we must proceed with increasing caution after having made the mistake.

After the first prescription has been made sometimes the patient will come to a standstill. The symptoms have changed in an orderly way; new symptoms have come up; but finally the symptoms have all retired in the reverse order to a former state and are hardly of sufficient importance to be considered. The patient will acknowledge that the troublesome symptoms have disappeared, and that he has little in the way of symptoms to report, but he does not feel well; there is no general sense of well-being, yet he can scarcely tell you why and where he does not feel well.

In such states we should wait until we are quite sure the remedy has ceased to act. There are remedies that have a "do nothing" stage in their unfolding, and we must be sure, before repeating the remedy, that the first prescription has entirely run out its cycle. If we have found a "do nothing" stage, it may be but a part of the remedy cycle; if so, the remedy is still acting and to repeat the remedy at this time could do no good and might do harm. In other words, this "do nothing" stage is an expression of the pathogenesis of the remedy as manifesting itself in the curative process, and by a little more patient waiting the patient will be ready for the next prescription. In these "do nothing" states no other remedy can fill in, because there are no strong indications for another remedy and the symptomatology has not altered to any marked degree except by lessening in intensity, and since there has been little change and no marked new symptoms have arisen, we have no guides for another remedy.

Then we must consider when to change the remedy for the second prescription. Besides the condition we have already spoken of, where new symptoms have appeared and there is an entire change, if the marked symptoms have disappeared and a new group of symptoms have appeared, with no relation to the former history of the patient, a new remedy must be considered.

Suppose in a chronic case these constitutional symptoms have been correctly met, and have gone through a range of potencies from the lowest up to the highest, and that they have all acted curatively, and the case has come to a standstill. After repeating the remedy we get no reaction. This constitutional remedy should be allowed to continue its curative action as long as it can be maintained and even if the symptoms have changed somewhat do not change the remedy as long as the patient shows improvement; but on the other hand, if the patient is not improving and there has been a change in the symptoms we can safely retake the case for the consideration of another remedy. We must make sure, however, that these symptoms are different from those the patient felt earlier, or have not been covered up by later developments, for a patient tends to become accustomed to certain symptoms and almost forgets that he has had them. If asked about them, he often replies that "they are nothing; he has always had them", but these may be an important part of the symptomatology and we may elicit the fact that these are just a return of old symptoms that have not been previously noticed or reported. On the other hand, it may be that we have really had all the action we can expect from the remedy that has been administered, and it is time to consider another remedy, since the first one has carried the patient as far as possible. A safe rule for procedure is: When in doubt, wait. In other words, never leave a constitutional remedy that has proven the simillimum for a considerable period, until you have extracted from it all the benefit that the remedy can contribute. Then, and only then, are you justified in changing the remedy.

It is quite possible that in making a second prescription we may find the simillimum to be complementary to the first. This is particularly well illustrated in the sicknesses of child life. There are often repeated tendencies for colds. The patient seems to be getting colds all the while, and a remedy like *Belladonna* may seem to be indicated and will cure the acute condition promptly. We may do this two or three times before we realize that these recurrences are an acute exacerbation of a chronic condition, and while *Belladonna* acts promptly and effectively, it is only because it is a complementary remedy to the underlying chronic *Calcarea* state. *Pulsatilla* may be as effective in acute manifestations while the constitutional condition calls for *Silica*. It is so with many remedies.

Then we may find constitutional conditions that require, for a complete cure, a succession of remedies, one remedy following another to good advantage. This may be a process of zigzagging a case to a cure because of lack of knowledge of our remedies or because the case does not unfold before us when we first consider it.

There is another possible reason for the successful succession of remedies. The first prescription may remove all the symptoms of one miasmatic condition, when suddenly a condition will arise which shows a basic condition of one of the other miasms. One miasm may have been submerged under another, and after the first has been removed by the simillimum, the second shows, and the plan of attack must be changed to include as weapons another group of stigmatic remedies. We cannot expect to eradicate any stigma with a single dose of any remedy, but we may so improve the manifestations that the underlying condition may show itself, perhaps later to return to the first miasm again.

In these chronic conditions, no prescription, either first or second, can be made without careful, thorough study of the case and the sequence of symptoms. It is only by working out the case with the repertories that we are able to see clearly the indicated constitutional remedy in the light of the symptoms that have been cured or relieved. It is only then that we can administer another remedy intelligently and with confidence (Roberts 1934).

4.1.3 Chatterjee

There is much to be learned from Roberts. What to do when the simillimum has been given? What to do with a partial cure? What to do with a partial cure plus new symptoms? When to change, when to repeat? But you see where he is coming from. He has understood the management of a case to be determined by his experience, and the 4th edition of the *Organon*. Chatterjee elaborates:

> An ideal homoeopathic treatment needs no second prescription. But in practice, the second prescription is a matter of every-day occurrence. The need for a second prescription arises on three accounts: (a) on drug account, (b) on physician account and (c) on patient account.

On drug account, it arises when the remedy, though selected on symptom totality basis with due regard to the patient's psycho-biographical history, has not acted or brought about cure; or when the cure is not complete and some symptoms still remain to be covered; or when the potency used falls short of the optimum for a cure.

On physician's account, the need arises when he has not correctly chosen the remedy with the inevitable result producing prolonged aggravation or when he confuses the case by burdening it with a number of ill-considered remedies, producing what is known as drug miasm.

On patient's account, the need may arise on several grounds, important of which are:

(1) When the first prescription has acted but further progressive relief is not felt.

(2) When a new set of symptoms, unrelated to the old, appears.

(3) When there is acute exacerbation of a chronic disease.

(4) When symptoms disappear but no relief is felt.

(5) When symptoms disappear against Hering's Law.

(6) When one of the three miasms, viz., psora, syphilis and sycosis is active either singly or in combination.

(7) When the disease has progressed from the functional stage to the structural stage, affecting the organs of the body.

It is essential that the changes in symptom occurring on above accounts are minutely observed and carefully analyzed before an attempt at a second prescription is made. A second prescription is not expected to act curatively, if the first has not acted as such. A bad first prescription can only lead to worse second prescription. There may be more than one prescription besides the first in the course of treatment, but all of them are regarded as second prescription because each one follows the preceding one and attempts to correct the existing symptoms.

There, is no third, fourth, fifth prescription in homoeopathy.

As will be seen from what has been stated above, cases of second prescription on drug account are really cases where the remedy has been correctly selected but fails to act or complete the cure. It fails to act because of the presence of miasm; it is unable to complete the cure because of persistence of certain symptoms inviting its complementary remedy to complete the job, or because of the low potency of the medicine which may require repetition either frequently in the same potency or at stated intervals in a higher potency. There will be occasion to touch upon these aspects when the most important of the three accounts, viz., the patient's account, is considered. The physician's account, on the other hand, is a distinct class by itself because of his causing the disease by his lapses in choosing the proper remedy in the course of treatment. If he detects his fault early, he has merely to antidote the medicine already given, take up the case afresh and select the remedy on right lines. But, if he has made a mess of the case by prescribing irrelevant remedies giving rise to drug-miasm, he has to take the help of such medicines as *Aloes* or *Nux-vomica* to prepare the ground for fresh case-taking and then proceed carefully as if it is a new case. For patients who have taken several inappropriate remedies, Dr. Kent has recommended *Calc., Ars., Sulph., Sep.,* and *Ip.,* whichever is relevant for tackling such cases.

Before a second prescription is made, it is the duty of a physician to satisfy himself that the remedy selected by him in the first prescription is the patient's similimum, that it has acted and that

(1) He is not repeating the remedy or changing its potency unnecessarily.

(2) He is not interfering with the remedy in the midst of its remedial action.

(3) He is not attempting to prescribe the remedy before the symptoms become stable.

(4) Good use of placebo has been made before his second prescription, allowing sufficient time to the first remedy to act and enabling any symptom-change to become stable.

The various methods of second prescription when the first remedy has been correctly selected and has acted are:

(1) Repetition of the remedy in the same potency or in higher potency.

(2) Remedy, complementary to the preceding drug.

(3) Cognate remedy.

(4) Antidote.

(5) New remedy.

(5) Low-potency remedy.

It needs to be pointed out in this connection that out of these six methods of second prescription, the first three methods viz., Repetition of Remedy, Complementary Remedy and Cognate Remedy, are available only when the condition of correctness of the first prescription is satisfied. The last three methods, viz., Antidote, New remedy, and Low potency remedy, however, are also available to meet situations other than those arising from correct prescribing. They are briefly discussed below :

Repetition of Remedy

The remedy is repeated in the same potency when the symptoms return but in a milder form. If the remedy is short acting, as in an acute case, it may be necessary to repeat the remedy as often as is necessary to cure the case. In a chronic case, where deep acting remedies are generally used, the repetition, under similar circumstances, has to be in a higher potency and at longer intervals. But care should be taken to see that some time-lag, say a week, is invariably allowed to confirm that the mild aggravation, when noticed in chronic cases, is not the "second aggravation" of Dr. Hahnemann. If it is a case of second aggravation. we may expect this to subside automatically in due course. No further medication in a higher potency is needed in such a case.

Even in an acute case, repetition in a higher potency is a necessity when the patient does not show improvement after the repetition of the remedy in the same potency.

Author's experience is that if a case, acute or chronic, needs repetition in the same potency, it avoids risk and produces better results when the remedy in the same potency is repeated through a complementary remedy or, where frequent repetition is deemed essential, the case is closed with a complementary remedy. Thus, in a case of *Aconite* fever, the case will be successfully closed if a dose of *sulphur* is given after remission of the fever. This will avoid any possible after-effects or return of the fever. Again, in case of flue-like fever with cold, cough, high fever, head and throat symptoms, *Belladonna* in alternation with *Arsenic alb.* either in the 6th or in the 30th potency will see the case through within 36 hours when given hourly, 2-hourly, 4-hourly or 6-hourly according to the severity of the case - the interval being increased with the progressive improvement of the case. This has acted almost as a specific in such cases and does not require more than 5 doses to bring about a complete cure. If this practice is followed, it should be assured that the remedies chosen are complementary and cover the symptoms.

Complementary Remedy

Very often it is noticed that even after prescribing the right remedy, the symptoms do not disappear wholly but continue in a mild form or reappear in a mild form after a temporary period of lull. Such cases require a more deep-acting remedy complementary to the first for a cure. It has been noted that during the period of dentition of children, some of them get fever and convulsion which, even after being remedied by *Belladonna*, reappear in some cases needing *Calcarea carb*, the deep-acting remedy complementary to *Belladonna* for a cure.

Cognate Remedy

Cognate remedies are remedies related in such a way that in the development of a disease when one category of symptoms is removed by the administration of a remedy, symptoms of its related remedy appear calling for its adoption. In complementary remedies, the character of symptoms remains the same, the difference is only in intensity; while in cognate remedies, a new category of symptoms, viz., that of the next related remedy, follows necessitating its prescription. It is not that in every case a cognate remedy is called for. In a case of cough ameliorated by cold drinks, *Causticum* alone will cure. But it might be that in some cases new symptoms such as sciatic pain of the left leg may appear requiring the help of its cognate *Colocynth* for a cure.

This cognate relationship is not restricted to two remedies only but extends to more than two. An example in point is the famous trio of Hahnemann-*Sulphur, Calcarea carb, Lycopodium* a very important combination, so helpful in treating chronic cold or in changing a constitution prone to cold. Another deep and long acting trio is *Sulphur-Sepia-Sarsaparilla* when it is sought to strengthen a weak and disease-prone constitution. It should be noted that there may be more than one cognate to a remedy as in complementary remedies, but the selection of the exact remedy will entirely depend on the symptom syndrome, after the first remedy had spent its force, allowing new symptoms to crop up. Cognate remedies are mostly used in treating chronic cases.

Antidote

"Antidote" is a very important and useful tool in the hands of a physician which can be used effectively both for defensive and offensive purposes - defensive, generally as a measure of countering the effect of wrong prescription and offensive, to cure the disease by fresh case-taking and seeking the correct remedy. Besides, there are many occasions when the effect of an acting remedy has to be antidoted in the interest of the patient. An antidote may take the form of prescribing the same remedy in a lower or a higher potency or it may be selected from the group of remedies already proved as such to the remedy in action. In all these cases, the decision has to be taken after carefully weighing the case under consideration, keeping in view the symptoms to he antidoted, the susceptibility of the patient and the condition of the vital force at the moment. While the remedy will depend on the symptoms, the potency will be determined by the susceptibility and the condition of the vital force. A case has to be antidoted:

(a) Where there is a severe aggravation of symptoms on continuing basis and the patient's life is in danger.

(b) Where the age and the condition of vital force cannot withstand the aggravation, though the remedy is the similimum.

(c) Where the structional change has advanced to a point of irreversibility.

(d) Where a completely new set of vexatious and distressing symptoms appears.

(e) Where the symptoms disappear but no relief is felt.

(f) Where the symptoms disappear against Hering's law.

New Remedy

Mere change of symptoms does not invite a new remedy. The more important consideration is the direction of cure, as pointed out by Dr. Kent. When a true remedy is administered, it brings change in symptoms - even old symptoms reappear, but the point to remember is whether the changes follow the

Hering's law. So long as it does, the same remedy should be allowed to act as it will bring about the cure. No new remedy is needed. But where the new symptoms show progressive aggravation of the disease and the patient feels worse, the case needs a new remedy based on the existing totality after a fresh case-taking with due regard to the past history and causation of the disease. If, however, the first remedy fails to act, even though it is the similimum or if after partial recovery new symptoms not accountable by the acting remedy appear, the presumption is that a latent miasm may have become active requiring the adoption of a suitable anti-miasmatic remedy which will remove the bottleneck and lead the case on the road of recovery. Very often, in a chronic case, new symptoms appear after the administration of a constitutional remedy but there is no apparent deterioration of condition of the patient. In such cases no new remedy need he given. The case has to be watched. The new symptoms are expected to vanish after a short period.

When a mixed miasmatic case has to be treated, the second prescription must, of necessity, be a new remedy. The first remedy is usually an anti-psoric remedy in such cases, as psora is the fundamental cause for any chronic disease. However, the rule, as pointed out in another connection, is to treat the active miasms first and, when its symptoms subside, treat the second which becomes active by then. When Psora is subdued with anti-psoric remedy and symptoms of sycosis come, e.g., corps of warts on face and hand, the next remedy to follow is anti-sycotic which is a new remedy involving also change in the plan of treatment from anti-psoric to antisycotic.

Low Potency Remedies

Low potency remedies are used as second prescription in incurable cases as and when the incurability of the case is confirmed by the first prescription.

A case is deemed incurable when the first prescription inspite of its being the similimum:

(a) does not evoke response from the patient and his condition continues to deteriorate;

(b) acts amelioratively only for a short time and then produces continuous aggravation of symptoms;

(c) acts adversely for a long period with aggravation of symptoms and continued deterioration of patient's health, and

(d) acts favourably with total disappearance of symptoms but this disappearance has not followed the Hering's law.

In all these cases, the true remedy fails to cure either because the vitality of the patient is too low or because there is an organic change and the change is such that its reversion to normalcy is impossible or because the structural change has progressed too far to retrace its step or because the body lacks some vital organ such as a lung or a kidney to make it not sufficiently responsive to the curative efforts of the medicine. The only way to treat such cases is to adopt palliative measures in the second prescription by prescribing remedies in the low potency on the basis of existing symptoms, taking every precaution that the case is not complicated by unimaginative repetition. Even then one has to be careful to see that *Ars., Apis., Kali-c., Sulph., Bacill.,*

Calc., Med., Phos., Sil., Tub. or constitutional remedies are not prescribed as they are likely to hasten the end. If, however, the existing symptoms do not allow selection of low potency remedies the case has to be given up as incurable under the homoeopathic system with such advice as is needed in each case (Chatterjee 2012).

4.1.4 Kent: The Second Prescription

There is a different tone here that is clear, directive and descriptive. Following on from this, is Kent's much more strident opinions in the *Lesser Writings*:

Editorial Note: What perplexing problems we often meet in practice! How we crave, at times, the advice of a master mind! We are so often the victims of prejudice, over-confidence or ignorance, and our patients suffer in consequence of this. Could we but understand the intricate laws governing the inner man, disease, and remedies, how much more wisely might we adjust ourselves to the far-reaching problems which endanger the life of a father, a mother, a noble son or an affectionate daughter. We would not then, as is so often done, impede or pervert the action of a carefully selected remedy by our impatience to get results, or by our impetuosity in hastening certain conditions which will not be hastened, or by our ignorance in so quickly changing remedies before one of them has had time for definite action. To help us in this noble work we reproduce below a masterly paper by Dr. J. T. Kent, read before the International Hahnemannian Association at Niagara Falls in 1888. - G. E. D.

What is more beautiful to look upon than the bud during its hourly changes to the rose in its bloom. This evolution has so often come to my mind when patiently awaiting the return of symptoms after the first prescription has exhausted its curative power. The return symptom-image unfolds the knowledge by which we know whether the first prescription was the specific or the palliative, i. e., we may know whether the remedy was deep enough to cure all the deranged vital wrong or simply a superficially acting remedy, capable of only a temporary effect. The many things learned by the action of the first remedy determine the kind of demand made upon the physician for the second prescription.

Many problems come up to be solved that must be solved, or failure may follow.

How long shall I watch and wait? Is a question frequently asked but seldom answered.

Is the remedy still acting? Is the vital reaction still affected by the impulse of the remedy?

If the symptoms are returning, how long shall they be watched before it is necessary to act or give medicine.?

Is the disease acute or chronic?

Why is the second prescription so much more difficult than the first?

Why is it that so many patients are benefited when first going to the physician and thereafter derive no benefit?

I presume that most good prescribers will say: "We have often acted too soon, but never waited too long." Many physicians fail because of not waiting, and yet the waiting must be governed by knowledge. Knowledge must be had, but where can it be obtained? To know that this waiting is right is quite different from waiting without a fixed purpose. This knowledge cannot be found where its existence is denied; it is not found with unbelievers and agnostics.

When the first prescription has been made and the remedy has been similar enough to change the existing image, we have but to wait for results. The manner of change taking place in the totality of symptoms signifies everything, yet the manner of the return of the image, provided it has disappeared, signifies more.

First. If aggravation of symptoms follow;

Second. If amelioration of symptoms follow;

1. Aggravation of existing symptoms may come on with general improvement of the patient, which means well; but

    If aggravation of the symptoms is attended with decline of the patient the cure is doubtful, and the case must be handled with extreme care, as it is seldom that such patients recover perfectly.

2. If amelioration follow the prescription, to what does the amelioration apply?

    It may apply to the general state or but to the few symptoms. If the patient does not feel the elasticity of life returning, the improved symptoms are the facts upon which to doubt recovery.

The knowledge that the disease is incurable often is obtained only in this way. In such cases every remedy may palliate his sufferings, but cure does not come. The symptoms that are the expressions of the debility are there, and hence the totality of the symptoms is not removed.

After the curative impulse has entirely subsided, the symptoms will appear one by one, falling into place to arrange an image of the disease before the intelligent physician for the purpose of cure.

If the first prescription has been continuously given, there has been but little if any chance of a pure returning image of the disease, therefore this image must be very unreliable.

When the remedy has been fully exhausted, then, and only then, can we trust the symptoms constituting the picture.

If the first prescription was the similimum, the symptoms will return and when they return-asking for the same remedy. Too often the remedy has been only similar enough to the superficial symptoms to change the totality and the image comes back altered, therefore resembling another remedy, which must always be regarded as a misfortune, by which the case is sometimes spoiled, and the hand of the master may fail to correct the wrong done.

Whenever the symptoms return the same image, calling for the same remedy, then it is that we have demonstrated, that-for a time, if the disease be chronic, we can but recommend the range of dynamics to cure this case. This rule is almost free from exceptions if the remedy is an antipsoric.

What must the physician do who has not the knowledge of dynamic medicines? He must sometimes see sick images come back without change of symptoms, though I believe it is seldom. The symptoms may call for *Phosphorus* as strongly as when he began, and *Phosphorus 6x* has served and no longer cures. What can he do but change his remedy? Can it be possible that man can be so ignorant of how to cure as to give a drug that is not indicated because the one that is indicated does not cure? These ignorant mortals condemn the system of Homoeopathy and feel that they have performed their duty to the sick, forgetting that ignorance was the culprit.

I have observed in cases where a low potency had been administered in frequently repeated doses, that some time must elapse before a perfect action will follow the higher potency; but where the dose had not been repeated after its action was first observed, the new and higher potency will act promptly. When the symptoms come back-after prudent waiting-unchanged, the selection was correct, and if the same potency fail to act a higher one will generally do so quite promptly, as did the lower one first. When the picture comes back unaltered except by the absence of some one or more symptoms, the remedy should never be changed until a still higher potency has been fully tested, as no harm can come to the case from giving a single dose of a medicine that has exhausted its curative powers. It is even negligence not to do such a thing.

Proper time to change

When the demonstration is clear that the present remedy has done all it is capable of doing and this demonstration can not be made until much higher potencies than usually made have been tried-then the time is present for the next prescription.

To change to the next remedy becomes a ponderous problem, and what shall it be?

The last appearing symptom shall be the guide to the next remedy. This is so whenever the image has been permitted to settle by watching and waiting for the shaping of the returning symptom-picture. Long have I waited after exhausting the power of a remedy, while observing a few of the old symptoms returning; finally a new symptom appears. This latest symptom will appear in the anamnesis as best related to some medicine having it as a characteristic which most likely have all the rest of the symptoms.

It is not supposed that this later appearing symptom is an old symptom on its way to final departure, for so long as old symptoms re-appear and disappear it is granted that no medicine is to be thought of.

It is an error to think of a medicine when a symptom-image is changing. The physician must wait for permanency or firmness in the relations of the image before making a prescription.

Some say, "I must give the patient medicine or he will go and see someone else." I have only to say that it were better had all sick folks gone somewhere else, for these doctors seldom cure but often complicate the sickness.

The acute expressions of a chronic disease have a different management from the acute disease, e.g., a child suffers from bronchitis in every change of weather. It may grow worse if treated with the remedy for the acute symptoms.

The miasm that predisposes the child to recurrent attacks must be considered.

One recently under my care had received *Antimonium tart., Calcarea, Sulphur, Lycopodium,* etc., in such indiscriminate confusion that the child was not cured. The waiting on *Sac-lac.* through several attacks permitted the drug-effects to pass off, and the true image of the sickness was permitted to express itself through several of the exacerbations taken as a whole.

When western ague is complicated with a miasm, a single paroxysm does not fully express the totality, but several must be grouped and the true image will be discovered. If the acute disease be complicated with a miasm the indicated remedy will wipe it out "cito, tuto et jucunde."

Avoid haste

All things oppose haste in prescribing. In very grave diseases haste is a common error, more frequently with the second prescription than the first. Many doctors suppose that a diphtheria demands a medicine immediately because "something must be done." This is an error; many a life has been saved by waiting and waiting.

For example:

A little girl was suffering from a severe attack of diphtheria and the mother had treated it four days with *Mercurius 3x*, and *Kali bich. 3x*, in alternation. She was poor, and therefore I did not refuse to take the case which was then in a very bad state: nose, mouth and larynx full of exudate.

After a long study the child received *Lycopodium CM*, one dose, dry, which cleared out the exudate from nose and fauces, but did not touch the larynx.

I dare not tell you how long I watched that child before I saw an indication for the second remedy which it would have needed had the *Lycopodium* been given when the child first took sick. I waited until the poor child was threatening dissolution when I saw a little tough yellow mucus in the mouth. *Kali bich. CM*, one dose, cleared the larynx in one day and there was no further medication necessary.

The first prescription is made with the entire image of the sickness formed. (People usually send for the doctor after there can be no doubt of the sickness to be treated.)

The doctor watches the improvement of the patient and the corresponding disappearance of the symptoms under the first prescription, and when the case comes to a standstill he is uneasy, and with increasing fidgetiness he awaits the coming indication for the next dose of medicine.

This fidgetiness which comes from a lack of knowledge unfits the physician as an observer and judge of symptoms; hence we see the doctor usually failing to cure his own children. He cannot wait and reason clearly over the returning symptoms.

While watching the prescriptions of beginners, I have observed very often the proper results of the first prescription. The patient has improved for a time, then ceased to respond to any remedy.

Close investigation generally reveals that this patient improved after the first dose of medicine, that the symptoms changed slightly without new symptoms, and the new "photo" seemed to call for some other remedy, when, of course, the remedy was changed and trouble began. Constant changing of remedies followed until all the antipsorics in the Chronic Diseases had been given on flitting symptom-images, and the patient is yet sick. This is the common experience of young Hahnemannians trying to find the right way. Some of experience make lesser blunders and some make few, but how many have made none? All of these blunders I have made, as I had no teacher, until I blundered upon the works of the great Master.

Wait and observe

The first prescription may not have been well chosen medicine, and then it becomes necessary to make a second effort.

As time brings about the re-examination of the patient, new facts are brought out in relation to the image of the sickness, indicating that the first medicine had not been suitable; perhaps several weeks have passed and the re-examination finds no change in the symptoms.

Shall I compare all the facts in the case to reassure myself of the correctness of the first prescription, or shall I wait longer?

Yes, to the former, of course, and if the remedy is still the most similar to all the symptoms, wait, and watch, and study the patient for a new light on his feelings to which he has become so accustomed he has not observed.

Commonly the new study of the case will reveal the reason why the first prescription has not cured: it was not appropriate.

If it still appears to be the most similar remedy the question arises: "How long shall I wait?"

At this point it should be duly appreciated that the length of time is not so important as being on the safe side, and "wait" is the only safe thing to do. It may have been many days, but that matters not, wait longer.

The finest curative action I ever observed was begun sixty days after the administration of the single dose.

The curative action may begin a slate as a long-acting drug can produce symptoms on a healthy body. This guide has never been thought of by our writers, but it is well to be considered. Why not?

It is the practice for some to go lower if a high potency has failed.

This method has but few recorded successes but should not be ignored.

The question next to be considered is the giving of a dose of medicine in water and divided doses. This has at times seemed to have favor over the single dry dose. This is open for discussion, requiring testimony of the many, not of few, to give weight.

The best reports are made from both methods, and both are in harmony with correct practice.

Improper action

The next important step to be considered is when the first prescription has acted improperly, or without curative results. Then it becomes necessary to consider a second prescription. The first prescription sometimes changes the symptoms that are harmless and painless into symptoms that are dangerous and painful.

If a rheumatism of the knee goes to the heart under a remedy prescribed for the one symptom, the remedy has done harm. It is an unfortunate prescription and must be antidoted. In incurable diseases when a remedy has set up destructive symptoms, an antidote must be considered.

If the remedy changes the general symptom-image, and the general state of the patient is growing worse, the question then comes up, was the prescription only similar to a part of the image, or is the disease incurable? Knowledge of disease may settle this question. If the disease is incurable, the action of the remedy was not expected to do more than to change the sufferings into peaceful symptoms, and the second prescription is to be considered only when new sufferings demand a remedy.

But suppose such a change of suffering comes after the first prescription and the disease is undoubtedly curable, then the conclusion must be that the first prescription was not the true specific, and that the true image has not been seen.

Wait until the old image has fully returned is all there is to do. It is hazardous practice to follow up rapidly all the changing symptoms in any sickness, with remedies that simply for the moment seem similar to the symptoms present. The observing physician will know by the symptoms and their directions, whether the patient is growing better or worse, even though he appear to the contrary to himself and his friends.

The complaints of patient or friends constitute no ground for a second prescription. The greatest sufferings may intervene in the change of symptoms during progress of permanent recovery, and if such symptoms are disturbed by a new prescription or palliated by inappropriate medicine, the patient may never be cured.

The object of the first prescription is to arrange the vital current or motion in a direction favorable to equilibrium, and when this is attained it must not be disturbed by a new interference. Ignorance in this sphere has cost millions of lives.

When will the medical world be willing to learn these principles so well that they can cure speedily, gently and permanently?

There can be no fixed time for making the second prescription; it may be many months.

The second prescription must be one that has a friendly relation to the last one or the preceding. No intelligent prescription can be made without knowing the last remedy. Concordances in Boenninghausen must not be ignored. The new remedy should sustain a complementary to the former.

Remedies suitable to follow

In managing a chronic sickness the remedy that conforms to an acute experience of the illness is worth knowing, as very often its chronic may be just the one that conforms to its symptoms.

Calcarea is the natural chronic of *Belladonna* and *Rhus; Natrum mur.* sustains the same relation to *Apis* and *Ignatia;* *Silicea* to *Pulsatilla; Sulphur* to *Aconite*. When *Pulsatilla* has been of great service in a given case and finally cures no more, while the symptoms now point to *Silicea*, the latter will be given with confidence as its complementary relation has long been established.

On the other hand *Causticum* and *Phosphorus* do not like to work after each other, nor will *Apis* do well after *Rhus*.

How physicians can make the second prescription without regard to the experience of nearly a century, is more than man can know.

These things are not written to instruct men of experience in the right way, but for the young men who have asked so often for the above notes of our present practice.

I am told almost daily that this kind of practice is splitting hairs, but I am convinced of the necessity of obeying every injunction.

Careful records

You should have no confidence in the experience of men who do not write out faithfully all the symptoms of the patient treated, and note carefully the remedy, and how given. Especially is this necessary in patients likely to need a second prescription.

The physician who has in his case-book the notes of every illness of his patients has wonderful hold of any community. He has the old symptoms and the remedies noted that cured, and he can make indirect inquiry after all the old symptoms long ago removed. The pleasure is not small found in consulting such a note-book.

Experience soon leads the close prescriber to note all the peculiar symptoms and to omit the nondescript wanderings indulged in by sick people; however, it is important to be correct in judgment.

Many physicians make a correct first prescription and the patient does well and cheers up for a while, but finally the test is made for the second and then all is lost. Homoeopathy is nothing if not true and, if true, the greatest accuracy of detail and method should be followed. It is fortunate that the physicians who repeat while the remedy is acting are such poor prescribers or their death-list would be enormous (Kent 1921).

4.1.5 Kent: What the People Should Know

These precepts, aphorisms, statements, comments and judgments contain years of clinical experience. He did not hold back in, *What the People Should Know*:

All who know and desire the benefits of the homoeopathic system of medicine, or art of healing, should acquaint themselves with the customs of the strict practitioners in order to avoid the deception of pretenders who are willing to imitate for diminutive fees, having no consideration for the patient nor the art of healing.

There are physicians who call themselves homoeopaths, but are so only in name, as they do not follow the methods worked out by Hahnemann. They give two medicines in one glass or alternate in two glasses, or in some cases give medicine in three or four glasses. They do not conform to Hahnemann's rules in taking the case and writing and preserving full records of the cases. The people who are acquainted with these facts cannot protect themselves against such impositions. The false and the true pervade all experiences and conditions of life, and the unenlightened and simple suffer by the deceptions of the false. The time has come when the followers of Hahnemann should furnish information to the people in order that they may recognize the genuine if they desire the benefits of the homoeopathic art of healing.

It should be known, first of all, that true homoeopathicians write out the symptoms of each and every patient, and preserve records for the benefit of such patient and the art of healing. A moment's thought must convince any person that human memory is too uncertain to be trusted with the long record of symptoms, even in a small practice; then how much more does the busy practitioner owe it to his patients to keep accurate records of their sicknesses? No physician is competent to make a second prescription if the symptoms upon which the first prescription was made have not been recorded with fullness and accuracy. Often in such a case the neglectful physician has forgotten the remedy given, even the one that has caused great improvement, but as there is no record of the case as to remedy or symptoms, and many of the latter have passed away, there is nothing to do but guess at a remedy, which generally spoils the case or so confuses it that the case seldom ends in a cure, and the sufferer always wonders why the doctor, who helped her so much at first, lost control of the case. Many cases that should end in perfect cure result in failure from the above negligence. Under such circumstances, when the physician has made a bad guess, he goes on spoiling his case by guessing and changing remedies to the disgust of the patient and injury to the art of healing. Such failure leads to the experimentation and temporizing which lead to disgrace. The people should be able to know whether a physician is what he calls himself, or is of another sect. The temptation is very strong to be "all things to all men."

The people should not expect to obtain homoeopathic results from a physician whose methods are not in accordance with the homoeopathic art of healing.

If a person wants mongrelism, regularism, polypharmacy, etc., by knowing the methods of the homoeopathist, he will be able to discriminate and select the kind of his preference, and it is reasonable to suppose that if he does not want a homoeopathist he will be glad to know how to shun him. Nothing is more humiliating to a Hahnemannian than to be called to the bedside and find that the people do not want him; but actually want one who gives medicine in two glasses because some old family doctor did so. Therefore, this information is as useful to him who would avoid a homoeopathist as to him who desires one.

Homoeopathic patrons going abroad and those far removed from their own physician, often ask for the address of a good Hahnemannian. Such address cannot always be given, yet there are many reserved, quiet Hahnemannian physicians scattered over the world, but they are sometimes hard to find. As far as possible, traveling homoeopathic patients should carry the address of Hahnemannians. In the absence of this a test may serve the purpose. Go to the most likely man who professes to practice after the manner of Hahnemann and tell him you want to consult him; but unless he writes out all the symptoms of the case as directed by Hahnemann, and continues to keep a record for future use, you cannot trust your case with him, as you have learned to have no confidence in the memory of the man. If he refuses to do this because of lack of time or ignorance, he should not be trusted, and it is best to bid him "good day" at once. If he be what he professes to be, he will be delighted to find a patient that knows so much of his system of practice, and the patient and physician will become fast friends.

There is another matter that the people should know about; that the homoeopathic physician cannot prescribe on the name of a disease; also, that names are often the cover of human ignorance; also, that two sicknesses of the same name are seldom given the same remedy. If a physician could prescribe on a name there would be no necessity to write out the many pages of symptoms that some long cases present.

The name of the disease does not reveal the symptoms in any case of sickness; the symptoms are the sole basis of the prescription; therefore it will appear that the name is not necessarily known, but the symptoms must be known to the physician in order that he may make a successful prescription. It will now appear that if a physician has not time to devote to the patient in order to secure the symptoms, he is likely to be just as useless to the patient as though he were ignorant, as he will, in either case, fail to procure the symptoms which are the only basis of a homoeopathic prescription. A little thought will enable a patient to ascertain whether this work is being done with care and intelligence or with ignorance, inexperience and laziness. It matters not from what excuse, if the physician fails to ascertain all the general and particular information in a case, he should not be trusted, as this labor, well performed, renders the rest of the work easy and a cure possible.

The people should also know that when such a record is on paper it is in such form that the patient may become the object of great study. In no other form can a likeness of his sickness be presented to the understanding of the true physician. Any physician who sneers at this plan shows how little he values human life and how much he falls short of a Hahnemannian.

The people should also know that the true physician may now compare such a record of facts with the symptoms of the Materia Medica until he has discovered that remedy most similar of all remedies to the written record. And when the patient has become intelligent, he will say to his physician: "Take your time, Doctor. I can wait until you find what you think is the most similar of all remedies, as I do not want to take any medicine you are in doubt about." This statement makes a grateful doctor, as he now knows that he is trusted and known, and has a patient intelligent and considerate. Under such circumstances the doctor can do his best and such patients obtain the best and uniform results.

People who are not thus instructed become troublesome to the physician, and even suspicious, when they need to inspire him with full confidence, and sometimes they even change physicians and do the one wrong thing that is against the best interest of the patient. It is possible and desirable for the people to be so instructed that they may select the safest physician and know when he is working intelligently. People who are instructed do not intrude upon the physician's sacred moments, but, on the contrary, aid him with trust and gratitude.

Only the ignorant suggest this and that in addition to what is being done, and the more ignorant the doctor the greater is the number of things resorted to, to make himself and others think he is doing something. The intelligent physician does what law and principles demand and nothing more; but the ignorant one knows no law and serves only his wavering experience, and appears to be doing so much for the patient, in spite of which the patient dies.

The physician must often long for a patient so well instructed as to say: "Doctor, if you are in doubt about what to give me, don't give me anything." Such words could only come from one who knows that there is a law governing all our vital activities, and that law must be invoked or disorder must increase to the destruction of all order in the human economy.

If it were not true that the human race is ignorant of the highest principles of science, mongrelistic medication could not find support upon the earth. It is true that if the people would study Hahnemann's *Organon* and thereby secure the safest medication for themselves and their families when sick, crude compounds and uncertain medication would not be the rule as it is at the present day. In all trades a man must be somewhat skillful in order to gain entrance to an intelligent patronage; but in the profession of medicine, personal tact excuses such lack of training and ignorance of all science of healing.

People who know what homoeopathy really is, should seek to introduce the principles among the most intelligent people by reading, and not by urging upon them a favorite physician (Kent 1921).

In these chapters and writings of Kent, we start to see his strength of uncompromising attitudes, his dogmatism, his obstinacy and his moral compass come through. And these writings also highlight his skill, the rosebud coming to bloom. There is so much of value in this chapter, precepts, aphorisms, statements, opinions, and forthrightness.

Whenever in doubt, wait.

1. *Always restudy your cases.*

2. *It is a rule after you have gone through a series of potencies, never to leave that remedy until one more dose of a higher potency has been given and tested.*
3. *Avoid haste*
4. *Keep careful records*
5. *Wait and observe*
6. *Did we mention – wait!*
7. *Wait some more*

For generations of prescribers, this advice has been that which was the basis, the solid foundation of their business, their thriving practice. It sets the tone for practice. These are sound principles on which to base great results. Nevertheless it is possible to see how Roberts, Chatterjee, Kent and others certainly strayed from the line in the 5th and 6th editions of the *Organon*. Again, the reason they have been quoted at length is not because they are right, in fact they are contradictory at times, but it is important to understand the landscape and determine just who said what and why. From that place the discerning reader can make up their own mind and create their own path.

Chapter Five | Observe, Understand and Act

In this chapter you will:
1. Learn the fundamentals of remedy reactions
2. Identify how authors changed their minds over time
3. Describe the various interpretations of different writers

Chapter 5

Observe, Understand and Act

5.1 Remedy Reactions

5.1.1 Hahnemann

Hahnemann changed his mind over time. Does this matter? Clearly he was getting some results with his early work. Clearly modern homeopaths following his 4th edition of the *Organon*, through the prism of Kent and Roberts, get results as well. But then so do those homeopaths using the 5th and 6th editions of the *Organon*. Does it matter? Ultimately? Really? It matters that practitioners understand what they are doing. And it certainly is imperative that teachers understand what they are saying.

> **Aphorism 157** But though it is certain that a homeopathically selected remedy does, by reason of its appropriateness and the minuteness of the dose, gently remove and annihilate the acute disease analogous to it, without manifesting its other unhomeopathic symptoms, that is to say, without the production of new, serious disturbances, yet it usually, immediately after ingestion - for the first hour, or for a few hours - causes a kind of

slight aggravation ['when the dose has not been sufficiently small and' in the Sixth Edition] (where the dose has been somewhat too large, however, for a considerable number of hours), which has so much resemblance to the original disease that it seems to the patient to be an aggravation of his own disease. But it is, in reality, nothing more than an extremely similar medicinal disease, somewhat exceeding in strength the original affection.

Aphorism 158 This slight homeopathic aggravation during the first hours - a very good prognostic that the acute disease will most probably yield to the first dose - is quite as it ought to be, as the medicinal disease must naturally be somewhat stronger than the malady to be cured if it is to overpower and extinguish the latter, just as a natural disease can remove and annihilate another one similar to it only when it is stronger than the latter (Paragraph 43 - 48).

Aphorism 161 When I here limit the so-called homeopathic aggravation, or rather the primary action of the homeopathic medicine that seems to increase somewhat the symptoms of the original disease, to the first or few hours, this is certainly true with respect to diseases of a more acute character and of recent origin, but where medicines of long action have to combat a malady of, considerable or of very long standing ...

It is important to note that this aphorism changed in the 6th edition. In the 5th edition of the *Organon*, Hahnemann advocates the use of the single dose:

where one dose, consequently, must continue to act for many days, we then occasionally see, during the first six, eight or ten days, the occurrence of some such primary actions ...

While in the 6th edition of the *Organon*, Hahnemann changes his perspective to advocate the use of repeated diluted doses:

> 'Where no such apparent increase of the original disease ought to appear during treatment and it does not so appear if the accurately chosen medicine was given in proper small, gradually higher doses, each somewhat modified with renewed dynamization (Paragraph 247). Such increase of the original symptoms of a chronic disease can appear only at the end of treatment when the cure is almost or quite finished'

Aphorism 246 was re-written in the 6th edition when Hahnemann was age 86 in Paris 1842, and published in 1921:

> "['Every perceptibly progressive and strikingly increasing amelioration during treatment is a condition which, as long as it lasts, completely precludes every repetition of the administration of any medicine whatsoever, because all the good the medicine taken continues to effect is now hastening towards its completion. This is not infrequently the case in acute diseases, but in more chronic diseases, on the other hand, a single dose of an appropriately selected homeopathic remedy will at times complete even with but slowly progressive improvement and give the help which such a remedy in such a case can accomplish naturally within 40, 50, 60, 100 days.
>
> This is, however, but rarely the case; and besides, it must be a matter of great importance to the physician as well as to the patient that were it possible, this period should be diminished to one-half, one-quarter, and even still less, so that a much more rapid cure might be obtained. And this may be very happily affected, as recent and oft - repeated observations have taught me under the following conditions: firstly, if the medicine selected

with the utmost care was perfectly homoeopathic; secondly, if it is highly potentised, dissolved in water and given in proper small dose that experience has taught as the most suitable in definite intervals for the quickest accomplishment of the cure but with the precaution, *that the degree of every dose deviate somewhat from the preceding and following* in order that the vital principle which is to be altered to a similar medicinal disease be not aroused to untoward reactions and revolt as is always the case* with unmodified and especially rapidly repeated doses.']

Foot note*

"What I said in the fifth edition of the *Organon*, in a long footnote to this paragraph in order to prevent these undesirable reactions of the vital energy, was all that experience I had justified. But during that last four or five years, however, all these difficulties are wholly solved by my new altered but perfected method. The same carefully selected medicine may now be given daily and for months, if necessary in this way namely, after the lower degree of potency has been used for one or two weeks in the treatment of a chronic disease, advance is made in the same way to the higher degrees, beginning according to the new dynamisation method, taught herewith with the use of the lowest degrees"

Aphorism 248 is re-written in the Sixth Edition:

"['For this purpose, we potentise anew the medicinal solution (with perhaps 8, 10, 12 succussions) from which we give the patient one or (increasingly) several teaspoonful doses, in long lasting diseases daily or every second day, in acute diseases every two to six hours and in very urgent cases every hour or oftener.

Thus in chronic diseases, every correctly chosen homeopathic medicine, even those whose action is of long duration, may be repeated daily for months with ever increasing success. If the solution is used up (in seven to fifteen days) it is necessary to add to the next solution of the same medicine if still indicated one or (though rarely) several pellets of a higher potency with which we continue so long as the patient experiences continued improvement without encountering one or another complaint that he never had before in his life. For if this happens, if the balance of the disease appears in a group of altered symptoms then another, one more homoeopathically related medicine must be chosen in place of the last and administered in the same repeated doses, mindful, however, of modifying the solution of every dose with thorough vigorous succussions, thus changing its degree of potency and increasing it somewhat. On the other hand, should there appear during almost daily repetition of the well indicated homeopathic remedy, towards the end of the treatment of a chronic disease, so-called (§ 161) homeopathic aggravations by which the balance of the morbid symptoms seem to again increase somewhat (the medicinal disease, similar to the original, now alone persistently manifests itself). The doses in that case must then be reduced still further and repeated in longer intervals and possibly stopped several days, in order to see if the convalescence need no further medicinal aid. The apparent symptoms (Schein - Symptom) caused by the excess of the homeopathic medicine will soon disappear and leave undisturbed health in its wake. If only a small vial say a dram of dilute alcohol is used in the treatment, in which is contained and dissolved through succussion one globule of the medicine which is to be used by olfaction every two, three or four days, this also must be thoroughly succussed eight to ten times before each olfaction.']

Chronic Diseases (Page 157)

"On any day when the remedy has produced too strong an action, the dose should be omitted for a day. If the symptoms of the disease alone appear, but are considerably aggravated even during the same moderate use of the medicine, then the time has come to break off in the use of the medicine for one or two weeks, and await a considerable improvement."*

*Footnote
On same method in acute diseases but give spoonfuls of the dilution every ½ hour or hour or 2 hour depending on the need."

"...but during the last years, since I have been giving every dose of the medicine in an incorruptible solution, divided over fifteen, twenty or thirty days and even more, no potentising in an attenuating vial is found too strong, and I again use ten strokes with each. So I herewith take back what I wrote on this subject three years ago in the first volume of this book on page 149 (Hahnemann, *The Chronic Diseases* translated by Tafel, published in 1896)."

5.1.2 Roberts

Roberts continues the thread in relation to remedy reactions in *The Principles and Art of Cure by Homoeopathy* (1936),

One of the first things required of a homeopathic physician is that his powers of observation shall be highly developed. His powers of discrimination should be very keenly attuned, first, that he may observe the patient in the analysis of the symptoms and the selection of the remedy, and second, that he may have the keen perception of the import of the symptoms after the remedy has been carefully selected and administered. After the administration of the simillimum some action should result. It is upon the development and interpretation of the action of the remedy, or the reaction of the vital energy to the remedy, that successful prescribing very largely depends.

What are we to expect after the remedy has been administered?

According to Hahnemann, the nearer similar the remedy the more reaction we may expect (*Organon*, 154, 155). If the exact simillimum is found we are apt to get a slight aggravation before relief comes.

On the other hand, if no changes take place, too long patient waiting is useless, for it is evidence that the simillimum has not been found; but the nearer the symptoms of the patient are to the symptoms of the remedy, the more sure we are to have some reaction. It is for us to determine what the reaction means and to interpret it in prognostic terms. We must be able to listen to the patient's report and from it and our powers of observation to determine what the remedy is doing. We know that when the remedy acts the symptoms will change, in either character or degree. There may be a disappearance of the symptoms, amelioration of the symptoms or increase of the symptoms, and these changes are the manifest action of the remedy on the vital energy or vital force; and it is these manifestations we must study.

Among the most common reactions after the remedy has been administered is aggravation or amelioration.

Now there are two types of aggravations, either of which may be manifest. There is the aggravation which is an aggravation of the disease condition, in which the patient grows worse. There may be a very different type of aggravation, in which the symptoms are worse, but the patient is growing better.

He will say, "I feel better, Doctor, but such-and-such symptoms are worse." The aggravation from the diseased state is an indication that the patient is growing weaker, and therefore the diseased state is growing stronger while his vital energy is ebbing.

On the other hand, the aggravation of the symptoms while the patient reports himself as feeling better is an indication that his vital force is being set in order, but individual symptoms may show aggravation.

We must also observe how the aggravation or amelioration occurs and the duration of these periods. In this connection we must always bear in mind that is the patient's welfare we are seeking, and it is for us to determine whether he is improving or declining. Sometimes he will say that he is weaker, yet on analysis of the symptoms you will find this is not true. The story of the symptoms is often of greater importance than the patient's opinion. After we have assured him of the amelioration of his condition and called his attention to the particular instances of improvement, he will better immediately.

An aggravation that is quick, short, and strong is to be desired, because we know that improvement will be rapid.

The repetition of the dose will be governed by the nature of the drug and the reaction of the vital energy. Some drugs, like Silica or Lycopodium, are slow in action and should be administered at long intervals, while others are quick to give a reaction and shorter in their duration. However, this is an absolutely dependable rule: NEVER REPEAT THE DOSE WHILE SYMPTOMS ARE MANIFEST FROM THE DOSE ALREADY TAKEN. This is the same rule applied to the proving as governs the administration of the remedy in the cure of sickness: NEVER REPEAT YOUR

REMEDY SO LONG AS IT CONTINUES TO ACT. The reason is as obvious in one case as in the other. It is absolutely essential to obtain a proving of real value and integrity as showing forth the characteristics of the drug and the order of the symptoms in their development.

Strictly speaking, the first prescription is the prescription that first reacts. A physician may make a mistake and not select a remedy that is similar, consequently with no reaction. Thus while we may seem to be looking for a second prescription, we are in reality looking for a first prescription to which the patient will react. In other words, the prescription must be considered as the simillimum. Unless the patient reacts to the administration of a remedy and it has produced an effect, it is not a true prescription, for it is quite evident that it is not the simillimum. It is really bungling.

In general, if the first prescription has had a beneficial reaction, that remedy should be allowed to complete its work to the fullest extent. In such conditions, the second prescription would be a repetition of the first; and since a remedy should not be changed without very good reasons, it is probable that the remedy may be repeated at the necessary intervals through a whole range of potencies, securing the full amount of good from each potency before passing on to the next.

The reaction to the correct prescription is that the striking features, the peculiar features, the concomitant symptoms on which the choice of the remedy was based, are the first symptoms to be removed; thus the guiding symptoms of the case have been obliterated. The picture has been almost erased, and only the trivial symptoms are left. Now if the remedy is repeated at this stage, the cycle of cure is broken; for the guiding symptoms will surely return only when the action of the remedy, the indications which give us the clue to our next step will present themselves. One of the hardest things for a physician to do is to keep his hands off at this stage. If the remedy is administered at this stage we will find an intermingling of drug symptoms, so that no intelligent prescription can be made.

A safe rule for procedure is: WHEN IN DOUBT, WAIT. In other words, never leave a constitutional remedy, that has proven the similimum for a considerable period, until you have extracted from it all the benefit that the remedy can contribute. Then, and only then, are you justified in changing the remedy.

It is quite possible that in making a second prescription we may find the similimum to be complementary to the first. This is particularly well illustrated in the sicknesses of child life. There are often repeated tendencies for colds. The patient seems to be getting colds all the while, and a remedy like Belladonna may seem to be indicated and will cure the acute condition promptly. We may do this two or three times before we realize that these recurrences are an acute exacerbation of a chronic condition, and while Belladonna acts promptly and effectively, it is only because it is a complementary remedy to the underlying chronic Calcarea state. Pulsatilla may be as effective in acute manifestations while the constitutional condition calls for Silica. It is so with many remedies.

Then we may find constitutional conditions that require for a complete cure, a succession of remedies, one remedy following another to good advantage. This may be a process of zigzagging a case to a cure because of lack of knowledge of our remedies or because the case does not unfold before us when we first consider it.

There is another possible reason for the successful succession of remedies. The first prescription may remove all the symptoms of one miasmatic condition, when suddenly a condition will arise which shows a basic condition of one of the other miasms. One miasm may have been submerged under another, and after the first has been removed by the simillimum, the second shows, and the plan of attack must be changed to include as weapons another group of astigmatic remedies. We cannot expect to eradicate any stigma with a single dose of any remedy, but we may so improve the manifestations that the underlying condition may show itself, perhaps later to return to the first miasm again (Roberts 1936).

5.1.3 Kent Prognosis after Observing the Action of the Remedy

Kent then provides us with his 12 remedy observations, relevant mainly for centessimal prescribing, one dose and wait. In *Prognosis after Observing the Action of the Remedy* (1900), he writes:

> After a prescription has been made the physician commences to make observations. The whole future of the patient may depend upon the conclusions that the physician arrives at from these observations, for his action depends very much upon his observations, and upon his action depends the good of the patient. If he is not conversant with the import of what he sees, he will undertake to do wrong things, he will make wrong prescriptions, he will change his medicines and do things to the detriment of the patient. There is absolutely but one way, and nothing can take the place of intelligence. If you talk with a great many physicians concerning the observations you have

made after giving the remedy you will find that the majority of them have only whims or notions on this subject and see nothing after the prescription is made. These observations I am going to give you have grown out of much watchfulness, long waiting and watching. If the homoeopathic physician is not an accurate observer, his observations will be indefinite; and if his observations are indefinite, his prescribing is indefinite.

It is taken for granted after a prescription has been made, and it is an accurate prescription, that it has acted. Now, if a medicine is acting it commences immediately to affect changes in the patient, and these changes are shown by signs and symptoms. The inner nature of the disease appears to the physician through the symptoms, and it is like watching the hands upon the clock. This watching and waiting and observing has to be done by the physician in order that he may judge by the changes what to do, and what not to do. It is true that the homoeopath is not long in doubt in many instances what not to do. There is always an index that tells him what not to do. If he is sharp and vigilant observer, he will see the index for every case. Of course, if a prescription is not related to the case, if it is a prescription that effects no changes, it does not take long to see what to do; much patient waiting for a foolish prescription is but loss of time, and that should be taken into account among the observations. The observations taken after a specific remedy has been given sufficiently related to the case to cause changes in the symptoms are those of value.

The changes are beginning, what are they like, what do they mean, to what do they amount? The physician must know when he listens to the reports of the patient what is going on. The remedy is known to act by the changing of the symptoms. The disappearance of symptoms, the increase of symptoms, the amelioration of symptoms, the order of the symptoms, are all changes from the remedy, and these changes are to be studied.

Among the commonest thing that remedies do is to aggravate or ameliorate. The aggravation is of two kinds; we may have an aggravation which is an aggravation of the disease, in which the patient is growing worse, or we may have an aggravation of the symptoms, in which the patient is growing better. An aggravation of the disease means that the patient is growing weaker, the symptoms are growing stronger; but the true homoeopathic aggravation, which is the aggravation of the symptoms of the patient while the patient is growing better, is something that the physician observes after a true homoeopathic prescription. The true homoeopathic aggravation, I say, is when the symptoms are worse, but the patient says, "I feel better."

We must now go into the particulars concerning these states as to the time and place, as to how the aggravation occurs, as to how the amelioration occurs, as to duration, etc. The aggravations and ameliorations, the directions of symptoms and many other things have to come up, and be observed and judgement has to be passed upon them.

First of all, the patient should be the aim of the physician, his whole idea should be centered upon the patient to determine whether he is improving or declining. We have to judge by the symptoms to know that this is taking place. Very often the patient will say, "I am growing weaker," and yet you may know that what he says is not true; so certainly can you rely upon the symptoms and their story, which is more faithful than the patient's opinion. Many times the patient will say, "Doctor, I am so much worse; " and yet your examine into his symptoms and you find that he is really doing very well. Just the moment that he finds out that you are encouraged, he feels better and rouses up and wants to eat.

By the symptoms, also, you can tell when the patient is really weaker and if the symptoms are taking an inward rather than an outward course you will know, even if he is encouraged, that there is no encouragement for him. We have in the symptoms that which we can rely upon. In the old school we have nothing but the information of the patient. This is of little account after making a homoeopathic prescription. The symptoms themselves must be corroborated. The patient's opinion must be corroborated by the symptoms. The symptoms do corroborate what the patients say in many instances, but the symptoms are the physician's most satisfactory evidence.

Another general remark needs to be made, namely, that we should know by the symptoms if the changes occurring are sufficiently interior. If the changes that are occurring are exterior, the physician must be acquainted with the meaning of them, so that he will know by that whether the disease is being healed from the innermost or whether the symptoms have merely changed according to their superficial nature. Incurable disease will very often be palliated by mild medicines that act only superficially, act upon the sensorium, act upon the senses, and, though the hidden and deep-seated trouble goes on and progresses, and is sometimes made worse, yet the patient is made comfortable. So that by the symptoms we can know whether the changes that are occurring are of sufficient depth, so that the patient may recover. The direction that the symptoms are taking is sufficient to tell that, especially in chronic disease.

A patient walks into the clinic, somewhat stoop-shouldered, with a hacking cough that he has had for a good many years. You judge by his looks that he has been sick a good while; his face is sickly, he is lean and anxious, he is careworn, he is suffering from poverty and poor clothing and scanty food. Now, you examine all of his symptoms, and they clearly indicate that he needs an antipsoric, for the symptoms are covered by an antipsoric, and from the history of the case you know he has needed it a good while. Upon prolonged examination, the antipsoric you have in mind is strengthened. You now examine his chest, and discover he has not the expansion that he ought to have, and you detect the presence of tuberculosis, and by feeble pulse and many other corroborating symptoms you ascertain that the patient has been steadily declining.

You give the medicine and he comes back in a few days with quite a sharp aggravation of the symptoms; he has an increased cough, he has a night sweat, and he is more feeble. Now, the homoeopathic physician likes to hear that; he likes to hear of an exacerbation of the symptoms; but this patient comes back in a week, and the aggravation is still present, and is somewhat on the increase, the patient is coughing worse, and the expectoration is more troublesome than ever, his night sweats have been going on; he comes back at the end of the second week and he is still worse, and all the symptoms have been worse since he took that medicine. He was comparatively comfortable before he took that medicine, but at the end of the fourth week he is steadily growing worse. There has been no amelioration following this aggravation, and he is evidently declining; he now cannot come to the office for he is so weak.

This, then, will be the first observation - a prolonged aggravation and final decline of the patient. What have we done? It has been a mistake, the antipsoric was too deep, it has established destruction. In this state the vital reaction was impossible, he was an incurable case. The question immediately comes up, what are you to do? Are you not going to give the homoeopathic remedy in such cases? The patient steadily declines. If you are in doubt about such action of the remedies and making the patient worse, you will probably have an undertaker's certificate to sign before long.

In incurable and doubtful cases give no higher than the 30th or 200th potency, and observe whether the aggravation is going to be too deep or too prolonged. There are many signs in the chest in such cases to make a physician doubt whether he will give a deep remedy when organic disease is present. Of course this does not apply when things are only threatening, when you have fear of their coming, but when you are sure of their being present. In the instance given has attempted to arouse his economy, but turned to destruction his whole organism. Then begin, in such cases, with a moderately low potency, and the 30th is low enough for anybody or anything.

When the patient does not seem to be quite so bad as the one I have just described, you get him a little earlier in his history before the trouble has gone quite so far, and then if you administer this same very high potency in the same way you will make a second observation. Though the aggravation is long and severe, yet you have a final reaction, or amelioration. The aggravation lasts for many weeks, perhaps, and then his feeble economy seems to react, and there is a slow but sure improvement. It shows that the disease has not progressed quite so far; the changes have not become quite so marked. At the end of three months he is prepared for another dose of medicine, and you see a repetition of the same thing, and you may know then that man was on the border land and had he gone further, cure would have been impossible. It is always well in doubtful cases to go to the lower potencies, and in this way go cautiously prepared to antidote the medicine if it takes the wrong course.

Then the second observation is, the long aggravation, but final and slow improvement. If, at the end of a few weeks, he is a little better and his symptoms are a little better than when he took the dose, there is some hope that finally the symptoms may have an outward manifestation whereby along with prolonged aggravations. You will find in such a patient there was the beginning of some very marked tissue change in some organ. We may know by observing the action of a remedy what state the tissues are in, as well as know something about the prognosis for the patient.

The third observation after administering the homoeopathic remedy is, where the aggravation is quick, short and strong with rapid improvement of the patient. Whenever you find an aggravation comes quickly, is short, and has been more or less vigorous, then you will find improvement of the patient will be long. Improvement will be marked, the reaction of the economy is vigorous, and there is no tendency to any structural change in the vital organs. Any structural change that may be present will be found on the surface, in organs that are not vital; abscesses will form and often glands that can be done without will suppurate in regions that are not important to the life of the patient. Such organic changes are surface changes, and are not like the changes that take place in the liver, in the kidneys, in the heart and in the brain. Make a difference in your mind between organic changes that take place in the organs that are vital, that carry on the work of the economy, and organic changes that take place in structures of the body that are not essential to life. An aggravation quick, short and strong is one that is to be wished for and is followed by quick improvement. Such is the slight aggravation of the symptoms that occurs in the first hours after the remedy in an acute sickness, or during the first few days in a chronic case.

Under the fourth observation, you will notice a class of cases wherein you will find very satisfactory cures, where the administration of the remedy is followed by no aggravation whatever. There is no organic disease, and no tendency to organic disease. The chronic condition itself to which the remedy is suitable is not of great depth, belongs to the functions of nerves rather than to threatened changes in tissues. You must realize that there are changes in tissues so marked that the vital force is disturbed in flowing through the economy, and yet so slight that man with all of his instruments of precision cannot observe them. Under such circumstances we may have sharp sufferings, but cures may come about without any aggravation. We know then that if there is no aggravation the potency just exactly fitted the case, but here you have a course of things that you need not always expect. Though there is nothing but a true nervous change in the economy after a potency that is not suitable, either too crude, or too high, for that patient, you will have an aggravated state of the symptoms. In cures without any aggravation we know that the potency is suitable, and the remedy, the curative remedy, provided that the symptoms go off and the patient returns to health in an orderly way. It is the highest order of cure in acute affections, yet the physician sometimes will be more satisfied if in the beginning of his prescribing he notices a slight aggravation of the symptoms. The fourth observation then relates to cases in which we have no aggravation, with recovery of patient.

The amelioration comes first and the aggravation comes afterwards is the fifth observation. At times you will see sickly patients, fully as sick as the one I mentioned in the first or second instance, walk into your office and after long study you administer a remedy. The patient comes back in a few days telling you how much better he was immediately after taking the medicine, and now he has three or four days of what appears to be a decided improvement, a prompt action of the remedy. The patient says he is better, and the symptoms seem to be better; but wait, and at the end of a week or four or five days all the symptoms are worse than when he first came to you. It is not a very uncommon thing in severe cases, in cases of a good many symptoms, to have an amelioration of the remedy come at once; but whatever you may say, the condition is unfavorable.

Either the remedy was only a superficial remedy, and could only act as a palliative, or the patient was incurable and the remedy was somewhat suitable. One of these two conclusions must be arrived at, and this can only be done by a re-examination of the patient and by finding out whether the symptoms relate to that remedy. Sometimes you will discover the remedy was an error; a further study of the case shows that the remedy was only similar to the most grievous symptoms, that it did not cover the whole case, that it did not affect the constitutional state of the patient, and then you will see that the patient is an incurable one and the selection was an unfavorable one. It is the best thing for the patient if the symptoms come back exactly as they were, but very often they come back changed, and then you must wait through grievous suffering for the picture; and the patient will wait better if the doctor confesses on the spot that his selection was not what it ought to be, and he hopes to do better next time. It is a strange thing how the patients will have an increase of confidence if the doctor will tell the truth. The acknowledgement of one's own ignorance begets confidence in an intelligent patient.

The higher and highest potencies will act in curable cases a long time. When I say act, I only speak from appearance; I should say they appear to act a long time, for the remedy acts at once and establishes a condition of order upon the patient, after which there is no use in giving medicine. This order will continue a considerable length of time, sometimes several months. The patients will get along just as well without any medicine, and get along better without that medicine that helped him than with it. In curable cases, whose prospects are good, they will go along for a long time, and become very much relieved of their symptoms. Now, if the patient comes back at the end of the first, second and third week and says he has done well, that he has been improving all the time from the CM of *Sulphur*, but at the end of the fourth week he comes back and says, "I have been running down," the physician must then pass judgment. Has this patient done something to spoil the action of this medicine? Has he been on a drunk? Has he handled chemical? Has he been in the fumes of Ammonia? No, he has done none of these things.

This condition is really an unfavorable one. To have a medicine act but a few weeks, whereas it ought to act for months thereafter, will make you suspicious of that patient. If nothing has taken place to interfere with this medicine in his economy you may be suspicious of this case.

This sixth observation is too short relief of symptoms. The relief after the constitutional remedy does not last long enough, does not last as long as it ought to. If you examine the third observation you find that there you have the quick aggravation followed by long amelioration; but in this, the sixth, you have the amelioration, but of too short duration. In instances where you have an aggravation immediately after, and then a quick rebound, you will never see, absolutely never see, too short an action of that remedy; or, in other words, too short an amelioration of the remedy. If there is a quick rebound, that amelioration should last; if it does not last, it is because of some condition that interferes with the action of the remedy; it may be unconscious on the part of the patient, or it may be intentional. A quick rebound means everything in the remedy, means that it is well chosen, that the vital economy is in a good state, and if everything goes well, recovery will take place.

In acute cases we may see this too short amelioration of the symptoms; for instance, a dose of medicine given in a most violent inflammation of the brain may remove all the symptoms for an hour, and the remedy have to be repeated, and at the end of that repetition we find only an amelioration of thirty minutes. You make up your mind, then, that patient is in a desperate condition, it is too short an amelioration. The action of *Belladonna* in some very acute red-faced conditions is instantaneous. In five minutes I have noticed the amelioration come, but the best kind of an amelioration is that which comes gradually at the end of an hour or two hours, as it is likely to remain. If it is too short an amelioration in acute cases, it is because such high grade inflammatory action is present that organs are threatened by the rapid processes going on. It is too short amelioration in chronic diseases, it means that there are structural changes and organs are destroyed or being destroyed or in a very precarious condition. These changes cannot always be diagnosed in life, but they are present, and an acute observer, who has been working earnestly for years, will often be able to diagnose the meaning of symptoms without any physical examination whatever, so that he can prophesy as to the patient. Such experiences of an intelligent physician in a family will cause them to look upon him as wiser than anyone else, for he knows all about their constitutions. This he acquires by studying their symptoms, the action of remedies upon them, and their symptoms after the medicines have been given. This enables him to know the reaction of a given patient, whether slow or quick, and how remedies affect each member of that family. This belongs to the physician, and he should be intelligent enough to know something about them when he has been treating them a little while. The old physician is in possession of this knowledge, while the student and the new physician have it all to learn.

Once in a while you will see a full time amelioration of the symptoms, yet no special relief of the patient, which is the seventh observation. There are certain patients that can only gain about so much; there are latent conditions, or latent existing organic conditions, in such patients that prevent improvement beyond a certain stage. A patient with one kidney can only improve to a certain degree; patient with fibrinous structural change in certain of places, tubercles that have become encysted and lungs capable of doing only limited work, will have symptoms, and these symptoms will be ameliorated from time to time with remedies, but the patient is only curable to a certain extent; he cannot go beyond and rise above such a state. Remember this after several medicines have been administered, and the amelioration of the case has existed often the full length of time of the remedies, but the patient has not risen above his own pitch in this length of time. The remedies act favorably, but the patient is not cured, and never can be cured. The patient is palliated in this instance, and it is a suitable palliation for homoeopathic remedies.

Observation eight. Some patients prove every remedy they get; patients inclined to be hysterical, overwrought, oversensitive to all things. The patient is said to have an idiosyncrasy to everything, and these oversensitive patients are often incurable. You administer a dose of a high potency, and they will go on and prove that medicine, and while under the influence of that medicine they are not under the influence of anything else. It takes possession of them, and acts as a disease does; the remedy has its prodromal period, its period of progress and its period of decline. Such patients are provers, they will prove the highest potencies. When you find a patient that proves everything you give in the higher potencies go back to the 30th and 200th potencies. Such patients are most annoying. You will often cure their acute diseases by giving them the 30th and 200th, and you will relieve their chronic diseases by giving them the 30th, 200th and 500th potencies. Many of them are born with this sensitivity and they will die with it; they are not capable of rising above this over-irritable and overwrought state. Such oversensitive patients are very useful to the homoeopathic physician. After they get out of one proving they are quite ready to repeat it or go into another.

The ninth observation is the action of the medicines upon provers. Healthy provers are always benefitted by provings, if they are properly conducted. It is well to observe carefully the constitutional states of an individual about to become a prover, and to write these down and subtract them from the proving. These symptoms will not very commonly appear during the proving; if they do, note the change in them.

The tenth observation relates to new symptoms appearing after the remedy. If a great number of new symptoms appear after the administration of a remedy, the prescription will generally prove an unfavorable one. Now and then the coming of a new symptom will simply be an old symptom coming up that the patient has not observed, and thinks it a new one. The greater the array of new symptoms coming out after the administration of a remedy, the more doubt there is thrown upon the prescription. The probability is, after these new symptoms have passed away, the patient will settle down to the original state and no improvement takes place. It did not sustain a true homoeopathic relation.

The eleventh observation is when old symptoms are observed to reappear. In proportion as old symptoms that have long been away return just in that proportion the disease is curable. They have only disappeared because newer ones have come up. It is quite a common thing for old symptoms to appear after the aggravation has come, and hence we see the symptoms disappearing in the reverse order of their coming. Those symptoms that are present subside, and old symptoms keep coming up. The physician must know himself that the patient is on the road to recovery, and it is well to say to the patient that this is encouraging; that diseases get well from above downwards, etc. Old symptoms often come back and go off without any change of medicine. It indicates that the medicine must be let alone. If the old symptoms come back to stay then a repetition of the dose is often necessary.

The twelfth observation. We will notice sometimes that symptoms take the wrong direction. For instance, if you prescribe for a rheumatism of the knees or feet, or for a rheumatism of the hands, and relief takes place at once in the rheumatism of the extremities, but the patient is taken down with violent internal distress that settles in the region of the heart, or centres in the spine, you see at once a transference has taken place from circumference to centre, and the remedy must be antidoted at once, otherwise structural change will take place in that new site. When diseases go from centre to circumference, going out from the centres of life, out from the heart, lungs, brain and spine, out from the interiors, upon the extremities, it is well. So it that we find most gouty patients get along best when their fingers and toes are in the worst condition. To prescribe for this, and see the heart symptoms grow worse is a most uncomfortable state of affairs, for it is attended with a gradual downward tendency. Eruptions upon the skin and affections in the extremities are good signs. I remember one time I was discharged from a violent old woman with quite a considerable amount of Billingsgate, who told me that when she called me in she could walk about, and now her ankles were swelled up with rheumatism so that she could not move. That patient got another doctor, but soon died. There is great danger in selecting a remedy on external symptoms alone, i. e., selecting a remedy that corresponds only to the skin and ignoring all the symptoms that the patient may have, ignoring the whole economy and general state of the patient; because it is true that that remedy that is related to the skin alone may drive in that skin disease and cause it to disappear while the patient himself is not cured. Such a patient will remain sick until that eruption comes back again or locates in another place (Kent 1900).

These then are Kent's famous 12 observations. Most definitely, Kent is writing about observations after a dry dose and waiting. This is essentially a style of prescribing after the 4th edition of Hahnemann's *Organon*. He elaborates in *The Second Prescription* (1900):

> The second prescription may be a repetition of the first, or it may be an antidote or a complement; but none of these things can

be considered unless the record has been again fully studied, unless the first examination, and all the things that have since arisen, have been carefully restudied that they may be brought again to the mind of the physician. This is one of the difficulties to contend with when patients change doctors, and one of the reasons why patients do not do well after such a change. The strict homoeopathic physician knows the importance of this and will try to ascertain the first prescription. If the former physician is strictly a homoeopathic physician, he is most competent of all others to make the second prescription. It is often a hardship for a patient to fall into the hands of a second doctor, no matter how much Materia Medica he may know. The medicine that has partly cured the case can often finish it, and that medicine should not be changed until there are good reasons for changing it. It is a very common thing for patients to come to me from the hands of good prescribers. I tell them to stay with their own doctor, I do not want them. Such changing is often a detriment to the patient, unless he brings a full record, and this is especially true in relation to a case that has been partially cured, where the remedy has acted properly. If the patient has no reasonable excuse to leave the doctor, it is really a matter of detriment to the patient for a physician to take another's patients at such a moment. It is not so much a question of ethics, it is not so much a question of the relation of one doctor to another, because friends can stand all that, but it is only after a tedious inspection of all the symptoms that an intelligent physician is capable of making a second prescription. As a general thing, if the first prescription has been beneficial it ought not to be left until it has done all that it can do. How is the second physician to know that? Then the duty of the physician is first to the patient, and to persuade the patient to return to his first doctor.

The rule is, after the first correct and homoeopathic prescription, the striking features for which that remedy was administered have been removed, a change has come, and the guiding symptoms of the case have been taken out, and only the common and trivial symptoms remain. It is true if the physician would wait long enough he would see the return of those symptoms, but usually when a patient walks into a doctor's office the doctor is in a hurry to make a prescription and does not wait until the proper time. He at once prescribes on the symptoms that are left, and this is one of the dangers to be avoided, a hurried second prescription. The patients are to be pitied that fall into the hand of such homoeopaths. Many patients are wonderfully benefitted by the first prescription; they have said to me "Dr. So and So benefitted me wonderfully for a while, and then he did not seem to be able to do me any good." The fact was that the first prescription was a correct one, having been properly chosen, and after that first prescription the doctor administered his medicines so hastily and so indiscriminately that nothing more was accomplished in the case. The trouble was that he did not wait long enough. It makes no difference whether the physician is so extremely conscientious that he does not want to give Sac. lac., or whether he is so ignorant that he does not know how to give it, the result is the same. The early repetition of the medicine and the continued giving of the same medicine, will prevent anything like an opportunity for the making of a second prescription.

If the doctor administers a well-chosen remedy, and repeats it too soon, he never gives the symptoms a chance to come back and call for a second prescription; but they become intermingled with drug symptoms, so that the rational second prescription cannot be made. The second prescription presupposes that the first one has been a correct one, that it has acted, and that it has been let alone. If the first prescription has not acted curatively, or has not been permitted to act the full time, it is impossible to get a second observation. The second observation is made when the case comes to a standstill, for after the first prescription has been made changes occur; there is a coming and going of symptoms, and while these changes are occurring no rational observation can be made of the case; if a second prescription be made during this time, it will be likely to spoil the whole case. If the patient is not given a perfect rest, if medicines are not kept out of the case, we will have no opportunity to make a rational second prescription. But if these precautions are observed, then we can really make an observation upon the return of the original symptoms, which is the first thing to be considered. Perhaps they are not so marked, but that is always the first thing to be looked for, the return of the original symptoms. While the confusion is going on after the administration of the remedy, while internal order is being established in the economy, we do not have the return of the original symptoms. This may be a matter of days, or weeks, or months, but if the return of symptoms is not observed what is there to be done?

Without symptoms what can the homoeopathic physician do? No matter what state the patient is in, what can the physician do without symptoms? There is no earthy guide to the remedy except by signs and symptoms. So that it is the duty of the physician to wait for the return of the original symptoms. If the symptoms return somewhat as they were, differing slightly in their intensity, increased or decreased, it is good. If the patient has not had these present symptoms for some time, if there has been a relief caused by the first prescription, and then the symptoms return some-what as in the original, this is one of the reasons for believing that the first prescription was a good one. If, after an interval of two or more months, the original symptoms return, we need very little information beyond this to know that the first prescription was a good one. In such a case when the symptoms return, when the patient has the same generals and particulars as formerly, it means that the first prescription was a good one, that the case is curable, and that the second prescription must be a repetition of the former.

Another reason for making a second prescription is the appearance of a lot of new symptoms taking the place of the old symptoms; the old symptoms do not return, but new symptoms come in their place. The patient says: "Well, doctor, you have cured me of those symptoms I had, but now I have these." The doctor, after examining carefully these new symptoms, immediately looks up the pathogenesis, and it is possible that he will find these symptoms in the drug that he had administered and then it looks like a proving. He asks the patient if he ever had these symptoms before. "Never to my recollection, doctor." Cross-examine him carefully to see if he is not mistaken, until it seems that they are really new symptoms. If so, the remedy has not acted properly. It was not homoeopathic to the case; and yet it was an unfortunate prescription, because it has caused the disease to progress in another direction, developing another group of symptoms.

This coming up of new symptoms means that they must be antidoted, if it is possible. The new symptoms combining with the old ones must be again studied and the second remedy must correspond more particularly to the new than to the old. It may cause the new symptoms to disappear and possibly have an effect upon the old ones. Any subsequent prescription takes into account all the things that have preceded it, all the conditions that have arisen, and, the third, fourth, fifth or sixth prescriptions have the same difficulties to surmount that are to be surmounted in the second. If the first prescription was an unfortunate one, then all the others are made with difficulty and fear.

It is rarely the case that a new prescription becomes necessary when the case merely comes to a standstill. The first prescription has been made and the symptoms commence to change in an orderly way; they change and interchange and new symptoms come up, but finally the symptoms go back to their original state, not marked enough to be of any importance, without any special suffering to the patient, and the patient has arrived at a state of standstill. The patient says, "I have no symptoms, yet I am not improving; I seemed to have come to a standstill position." He says this as to himself, not as to the symptoms. He has come to a standstill.

It is the duty of the physician then to wait, and wait a long time, but if after many months no outward symptoms have appeared, no external tendency of the disease, it is true that another dose of the same medicine will not do harm and the same remedy is the only one that can be considered. A new one cannot be entertained, because there is no guide to it; but another dose of the same medicine can cause the patient to be jogged along the way of feeling better, but there should never be any haste about it. Wait a long time when patients come to a standstill; but when, as in the first instance, the return of the original symptoms is observed, then you have some guide to the administration of the medicine.

The second prescription, then, technically speaking, is the prescription after the one that has acted.

You may administer a dozen remedies without having any effect upon the economy, and yet no prescription has been administered that has been specific. You may fool away much time in administering remedies that are not related to the case. The result is the same. Consider the first prescription the one that has acted, that one that has effected changes, and subsequent to that the next prescription is the second.

The next thing we have to consider is the change of the remedy in a second prescription. Under what circumstances must we change the remedy? One instance I have mentioned, when striking new symptoms appear, and there is an entire change of base in the symptoms, so that the headache, perhaps, which has lasted a long time, disappears. After the administration of the medicine, when a new group of symptoms appears somewhat in the body relative to the patient, such as the patient has never had, this new group of symptoms means that a new remedy must be considered, and under such circumstances the change of the remedy will be the second prescription, and the second prescription in this case calls for a change of remedy.

We will suppose another instance where the remedy must be changed. A patient has been for years under treatment for a constitutional chronic disorder, and you have gone through the potencies ranging from the lowest to the highest, and they have acted curatively. You have administered the different potencies, repeating the same potency until it would not act any longer, and then going higher, until you have gone through the whole range of potencies. You can repeat that remedy many times on a paucity of symptoms, when you cannot give another remedy, simply because it has demonstrated itself to be the patient's constitutional remedy. This remedy should not be changed so long as the curative action can be maintained. Even if the symptoms have been changed do not change the remedy, provided the patient has continuously improved. If the patient says he has improved continuously, and though it would be impossible for you, at this date, from the present symptoms, to select that remedy, hold on to that remedy, so long as you can secure improvement and good from it, though the symptoms have changed. Many physicians say: "If the symptoms change, I change the remedy." That is one of the most detrimental things that can be done. Change the remedy if the symptoms have changed, providing the patients has not improved; but if the patient has improved, though the symptoms have changed, continue that remedy so long as the patient improves. Very often the patients are giving forth symptoms long forgotten. The patient has not heard them, or has not felt them, because he has become accustomed to them, like the ticking or the striking of the clock on the wall. Many of the symptoms that appear, and the slightest changes that occur, are old symptoms coming back. The patient is not always able to say that they are old symptoms returning, but finally the daughter or somebody in the house will delight you by saying that her mother had these things years ago and she has forgotten them. This is likely to be the case whenever a patient is proving. So long as curative action can be obtained, and even though the symptoms have changed, provided the patient is improving, hands off. Whenever in doubt, wait. It is a rule after you have gone through a series of potencies, never to leave that remedy until one or more dose of a higher potency has been given and tested. But when this dose of a higher potency has been given and tested, without effect, that is the only means you have of knowing that this remedy has done all the good it can for this patient and that a change is necessary.

There is another instance to be spoken of, and that is when the second prescription becomes a complementary one. A second prescription is sometimes necessary to complement the former and this is always a change of remedy. Suppose a little four or five year old child, a large-headed, bright, blue-eyed boy, is subject to taking cold, and every cold settles in the head with flushed face and throbbing carotids, etc., you say give him *Belladonna* and *Belladonna* relieves, but it does not act as a constitutional remedy. He continues to have these headaches, which are due to a psoric constitution, and the time comes when *Bell* will not relieve them; but upon a thorough study of the case, you find that when his symptoms are not acute, when he does not have his cold and fever, he does not have the headache and you see an entirely different remedy indicated. You study over the flabby muscles, and you find his glands are enlarged; that he takes cold with every change in the weather, like enough he craves eggs, and you decide that the case calls for *Calcarea*. The fact that *Bell.* was so closely related to him and only acted as a palliative further emphasizes it. It is a loss of time to treat more than the first or second acute paroxysm. Do not give *Calcarea* during the paroxysm, but after the wire edge has been rubbed off by *Bell.* give him that constitutional remedy that is complementary to *Bell*, which is *Calcarea*. Many remedies associate after this fashion.

Then there are series of remedies, as, for instance, *Sulphur, Calcarea* and *Lycopodium*. A medicine always leads to one of its own cognates, and we find that the cognates are closely related to each other, like *Sepia* and *Nux Vomica*. A bilious fever in a *Sepia* constitution is likely to call for *Nux*, and as soon as that bilious fever or remittent fever has subsided the symptoms of *Sepia* come out immediately, showing the complementary relation of *Nux* and *Sepia*. If the patient has been under the influence of *Sepia* some time, and comes down with some acute inflammatory attack, he is very likely to run towards *Nux* or another of its cognates. The whole Materia Medica abounds with these complementary and cognate relationships.

The second prescription also takes into consideration the change of plan of treatment. The plan of treatment consists in assuming that the case is a psoric one, if looming up before the eyes, all the symptoms in the case and its history indicate psora. The treatment has probably consisted of *Sulphur, Graphites* and such medicines as are well known to be antipsoric. The symptoms have run to these remedies; but, behold, after you have made the patient wonderfully well, and you have effected marked changes in his system, so that the psoric symptoms have disappeared, he comes into your office with an ulcerated sore throat, with dreadful head pains and with the constitutional state and appearance that will lead you to say, "My dear sir, did you ever have syphilis?" "Yes, twenty or thirty years ago, and it was cured with Mercury." Now, the psoric condition has been subdued and this old syphilitic condition has come up. This, then indicates a second prescription. You have to adjust your remedies to an entirely new state of things. So it is also with regard to sycosis; these states may alternate with each other. When one is uppermost, the other is quiet, so you have to change your plan of treatment according to the state of the patient.

No prescription can be made for any patient except after a careful and prolonged study of the case, to know what it promises in the symptoms, and everything that has existed previously. That is the important thing. Always restudy your cases. Do not administer a medicine without knowing the constitution of the patient, because it is a hazardous and dangerous thing to do (Kent 1900).

Chapter Six | Specific Techniques

In this chapter you will:

1. Identify the different techniques advocated by various writers
2. Understand Vithoulkas's directives
3. Grasp their advantages and limitations

Chapter 6

Specific Techniques

6.1 When This Happens ... Do That

With the literature explored and integrated, there remain some practicalities to discuss. When it comes to understanding a remedy reaction, what do we do in any given situation? When do we change the medicine?

6.1.1 Sherr

Jeremy Sherr is a contemporary homeopathic educator who places an emphasis on the second prescription and understanding the reaction of the remedy. I found it valuable to hear this (paraphrased by me below) in his postgraduate courses. He argues that there are in fact only four remedy responses:

1. Nothing happens.
2. It's all good.
3. It's all bad.
4. Some good things and some bad things happen.

There is an elegant simplicity to this formula. Although seemingly simple, it's also deserving of more in-depth investigation.

Nothing Happens | No Change

Why is it that nothing happens? Actually there are 10 possible reasons:

1. Imperfect similar.
2. Imperfect potency.
3. The remedy has been antidoted.
4. The patient is insensitive.
5. The patient hasn't taken the remedy.
6. The patient hasn't been compliant with the instructions for taking the remedy.
7. The patient hasn't observed any changes that have taken place.
8. The remedy is slow acting.
9. Obstacles to cure are impeding the action of the remedy.
10. Remedy not succussed in between each dose.

In clinical practice, one of the previous reasons can happen a lot of the time, and how you act after determining why nothing has happened is important.

Reason	Action
Imperfect similar	Re-take the case and find a closer simile, or better still the simillimum
Imperfect potency	Give another potency
Remedy has been antidoted	Give the same remedy again

Specific Techniques

Patient is insensitive	Give another clearly indicated remedy before determining that homeopathy is unsuitable
Patient hasn't taken the remedy	Determine the reason. Was it fear, anxiety, possibly stubbornness? Ask the patient to take the remedy while in your office or find some alternative health care arrangements
Patient isn't compliant with instructions for taking the remedy	Encourage the patient to either take the remedy as directed or find some alternative health care arrangements
Patient hasn't observed any changes that have taken place	Determine with careful questioning if any even imperceptible changes have taken place
Remedy is slow acting	Wait and allow the remedy more time to act
Obstacles to cure impeding the action of the remedy	Negotiate with the patient to do your best to work around the obstacles
Remedy not succussed in between each dose	Show the patient how to succuss the remedy, and get the patient to take the remedy while still in your office

Note: it does not matter if you have prescribed by the 4th, 5th or 6th edition of the *Organon*, the principles here are the same.

The Total Positive Reaction

The patient experiences improvement in all areas.

Action: Do nothing. Wait. Relax. Repeat only when symptoms return; when it is clear that the vital force has gotten the message. Change the remedy only when it is very clear the whole symptom picture has changed. Only if necessary this second remedy will often be a complementary remedy to the first remedy. It is a sound working principle to be available for the patient for a quick phone call to help compliance or persuade the patient to wait before repeating the medicine.

Note: Does not matter if you have prescribed by the 4th, 5th or 6th edition of the *Organon*.

The Total Negative Reaction

The patient experiences worsening of symptoms in all areas. If this is during or soon after the remedy is taken, it may be an aggravation or a proving reaction. If it is 4-6 weeks after the last dose, it is rare. It may indicate that the patient has a very low vital force and/or is incurable (according to Vithoulkas and Kent).

Action: Carefully study your case notes to determine if it is an aggravation of existing symptoms or a proving reaction. If the patient is experiencing true aggravation of symptoms, wait and manage the patient through the aggravation. Talk to the patient to manage expectations and ease anxiety during the symptoms. If the patient is experiencing a proving reaction, retake the case.

Note: It does not matter if you have prescribed by the 4th, 5th or 6th edition of the *Organon*.

The Partially Positive and Negative Reaction

This reaction is where it gets interesting, and is a staple of daily practice. How you, as a practitioner handle this situation will determine how busy your clinic will be. There are some useful tricks, tools and tips that can assist. Learning how to deal with one-side cases is crucial (see the later chapter). In addition, understanding Hahnemann's guidelines for treating cases with clear characteristic symptoms but not enough remedies is crucial (see later chapter).

Action: Refer to the best literature on this daily reality found in one of the following books:

1. Kent, *Lectures on Philosophy*, p.253

2. Roberts, *Principles,* p124-125
3. Hahnemann, *Chronic Diseases,* p199
4. Vithoulkas, *Science of Homeopathy,* Ch 15 and Appendix B

Memorise the 12 observations of Kent, rely on the 22 observations by Vithoulkas or read de Schepper (2004). Understand and identify the contexts in which each of these books can be the most useful. A summary of potentially useful reference books is included next:

6.1.2 Vithoulkas

Vithoulkas's appendix B in the *Science of Homeopathy* (1980) is a gem and it should be read, re-read, understood and integrated by every homeopath. There is such value in learning his graphs. There is very little if anything that can happen in practice that is not there, with a clear explanation and action plan.

Disadvantages of the Graphs

Unfortunately the graphs that he devised are limited to a Kentian prescription style of one dose and wait for a month, and so from that perspective are limited in value. However, many of the directives that he gives often hold good for all types of prescribing, whether it is once a day or twice a day, or as he seems to do and advocate in the book, once a month or so. Many times I have referred to the back of the book to get its advice on what he feels is going on when a patient reacts in a very specific way.

6.1.3 Henriques

There have been other attempts at creating clarity. Nicola Henriques has written an excellent book on the second prescription called *Crossroads to Cure* (1998). Henriques delivers essentially a Kentian approach to case management and the advice is measured, excellent and deserves meticulous reading.

6.1.4 De Schepper

In *Achieving and Maintaining the Simillimum* (2004), de Schepper gives excellent advice about the use of the Q potencies in particular and how to manage those. To quote a recent graduate,

> During school, his books were my go-to books for posology and case management. Before I read them on my own out of curiosity, I had no clue that there were such fundamental differences between the 4th, 5th and 6th editions of the *Organon*, and had to identify for myself that I was being taught from a 4th edition perspective. I had many 'aha' moments after reading this book, and the other two in this series.

He makes an all encompassing attempt to integrate the 4th, 5th and 6th edition prescribing style in his diagrams and explanations.

6.1.5 Summary and Collective Wisdom

1. The simillimum does nothing new.
2. If something new happens, it is not the simillimum.
3. If it is a one-sided case, then we reanalyse the new auxilliary symptoms with the existing to form a new simillimum picture.
4. Never prescribe when the previous dose is still acting.
5. Never hit a rolling golf ball.

Chapter Seven | Repetition of the Dose

In this chapter we:

1. Review the literature
2. Learn the rules of repetition from the masters of homeopathy
3. Identify their points of difference and similarity

Chapter 7
Repetition of the Dose

7.1 4th edition of the *Organon* – Opinions

When shall the second remedy be given? After the first is extinguished.

7.1.1 Hussey

It's simple. Hussey elaborates;

> I am well aware that I can give you nothing that is new on this subject. The method of making the homeopathic prescription was fully worked out by Samuel Hahnemann and was elaborated by his immediate followers. And such was the remarkable skill and insight with which it was done that now with the great strides which in many ways have been made in medicine, no improvement upon their method has been made. Consequently I can give you what I have found in Hahnemann's *Organon* and *Chronic Diseases* and in the writings of Bönninghausen.
>
> As the subject, "the second prescription", has not been written about in medical journals nor discussed in medical societies enough to become hackneyed, a review of it here will not be amiss. We are conversant with what constitutes the essentials for

the homeopathic prescription: with the painstaking study of the patient: his idiosyncrasies; environment; occupation; habits of life; and of everything which may be the cause of, or contribute to, his ailment and must be eliminated as the first step towards restoring him to health. And, finally, of the careful summing up of every abnormal thing which his case presents as the "totality of the symptoms".

After all of this has been mastered comes the selection of the curative homeopathic remedy, based upon the knowledge of the effects of drugs upon the healthy system and applied by selecting for administration the drug whose action on the healthy is most like the diseased condition of the patient. When all of this is done we are, perhaps, apt to feel that we have mastered the essentials of the case, and have got it well started on the way to cure. But it is a fact that then, often the treatment has only just begun. The second prescription is no whit less important, calls for no less study, critical analysis and discerning judgment than the first: and upon it depends no less the perfect cure. The making of the second prescription is often more difficult, even, than the first. The first is made, usually with the clear image of the patient and his disease for guidance. In the second, all of that plus the effect of the first must be considered. Before the second comes, there must be the watching of the effect of the first, the development of the case under treatment, and the determining of when the second shall be given, as well as what it shall be. It would seem that all that would be necessary to do would be to follow the rule and, noting all of the symptoms presented, apply the simillimum. But to carry these rules out in practice requires an understanding and interpretation which is somewhat complex.

The first consideration is that of time. When shall the second prescription be given? Hahnemann's rule regarding that is very explicit and a century of experience has proved its value. The time for considering the second prescription is when it is clear that the first has done all for the patient that it is capable, in any potency, of doing.

Hahnemann mentions three great mistakes which the homeopathic physician cannot too carefully avoid. These precautions should be printed and posted in every physician's office. They are, first, to suppose that the doses that his experience and observation induced him to adopt are too small. Second, is the improper use of a remedy. And the third consists in not letting the remedy act a sufficient length of time. This he considered a great mistake: and he emphatically asserts that the homeopathic physician cannot too carefully avoid the too hasty repetition of the remedy.

Particularly in chronic diseases, giving the remedy in the proper potency in the first prescription, and the cessation of its administration when improvement has surely begun, is as essential to the accuracy of the second prescription as any feature of the case. The first prescription must not confuse the case. It cannot fail to do so if it is given in such strength as to produce drug symptoms, or if its administration is continued after improvement has become established. It is very evident that, if the patient's symptoms are mixed and confused with drug symptoms, the physician lacks the information upon which to base a new prescription. Such a case presents an almost hopeless problem to the prescriber. And such a course has spoiled many a brilliant cure.

In chronic cases, if the remedy has acted favorably within the first eight or ten days, it is a sure indication that it is the right remedy. But, because it has done so, it must not be supposed that it can act no more without repetition. It often takes forty or even fifty days for some of the great antipsoric remedies to complete their action, and it would be the greatest unwisdom to give another remedy before the lapse of that time. And even then it is not always, nor even often, that another remedy must be given immediately. The surest and safest way is to let the remedy act as long as the improvement of the patient continues, even if it be an indefinite time. Many times such improvement continues to the complete restoration to health. He who observes this rule with the greatest care will be the most successful homeopathic prescriber.

The whole case fails if the antipsoric remedy which has been prescribed is not permitted to act uninterruptedly to the end. The failure to do this is the principle reason why so many patients are benefited when first going to a physician, and afterward fail to improve.

Another thing to keep in mind to avoid confusing the second prescription is the fact that a remedy which is not strictly homeopathic to the case may change the symptoms of the patient. So the prescriber must be careful to note whether any new symptoms belong particularly to the medicine given. That point, of all the rules laid down for guidance to the second prescription, is the most difficult to discern.

For if a remedy is given which is homeopathic to the case, all of the new symptoms arising in its development are likely to resemble the remedy. In noting the effects of medicines and the changes of symptoms under prescription, it is an aid to prognosis to remember that if the more troublesome symptoms of the patient are aggravated, and there is also a general improvement, the prescription is probably correct, and cure will follow. But if with aggravation of the more superficial symptoms the patient becomes generally worse and declines, either the remedy is not strictly homeopathic or the patient cannot recover. And so with the amelioration of symptoms. If with it there is a general improvement and sense of general well-being, the prescription is correct and the patient will undoubtedly recover. I have many times found it to be the case that if my most careful prescribing would simply relieve the most distressing symptoms, they being followed by others which in turn might be relieved, and the patient not improve generally, I could safely give an unfavorable prognosis.

When the first prescription was the simillimum, and yet was not capable in the form given of completing the cure, the same original symptoms will return and will call for the same remedy for the second prescription. In such a case it will usually be best to give it in a higher potency. But, if the symptoms change and new ones appear, and the first prescription was not incorrect nor too strong, nor continued too long, then another remedy must be considered. But here haste must be avoided. It is better to wait until the new symptoms have developed so as to make the prescription sure: then the rule to be followed must be the same as for the first prescription. It is very necessary in making the second prescription that the physician should know what the symptom-picture of the case was before the first prescription was given, and what the first prescription was. If the first one was not the proper one, and is doing harm, it must be antidoted, and the physician must wait until the original picture of the disease returns. Only thus can an intelligent prescription be made.

The character of the case in regard to acuteness must be considered in determining the time for giving a new remedy. As a rule acute diseases call for short-acting remedies and chronic diseases for those which act longer and which are capable of affecting the system in the most profound manner. But the action of even the antipsoric remedies is proportionate to the acute or chronic character of the disease. Consequently the character of the disease determines the time for the second prescription, rather than the possibilities of the action of the remedy.

One other important thing must not be neglected: that is, the relationship the proposed new remedy bears to the one already given. It must be complementary to it; or one which follows it well. That is more important than is always appreciated. Early in my practice, one who knew the work of Constantine Hering well told me that the first question he asked when seeing a case in consultation was. "What medicine has the patient been taking?" His first requisite for a new prescription was a knowledge of what had gone before. The subject of drug relationship was very fully worked out and given in Boenninhausen's Therapeutic Pocket-book. It is given more conveniently accessible in Knerr's Repertory to Hering's Guiding Symptoms.

There it is grouped under six heads:

Antidotes. To the effects of molecular and massive doses: chemical antidotes to poisoning: to the lasting or chronic effects super induced by the drug.

Collateral. Side relations (congenors) belonging to the same or allied botanical family or chemical groups.

Compatible. Drugs following well.

Complementary. Supplying the part of another drug.

Inimical. Drugs disagreeing; incompatible; do not follow well.

Similar. Drugs suggested for comparison by reason of their similarity; usually compa ible, unless too similar; like *Nux vomica* and *Ignatia*.

I think that what I have related will not lessen your appreciation of the difficulty of making a homeopathic prescription. But, as one of our great teachers aptly says, "Homeopathy is nothing if not true; and, if true, the greatest accuracy of detail and method should be followed."

I have heard it questioned whether a method that requires and involves so much is really worth while. The answer to that is short if one aims to fulfill his mission and heal the sick. But there are many things working against the adoption of homeopathy to the extent it deserves. It is not within the province of this paper to enumerate them: but I may be excused if I mention a potent one. That is the demand of the age for speed. Everywhere, even where it is not necessary, is the mad spirit of haste. The demand is for short cuts - too often at the expense of permanent welfare. But nature's processes are what they are; not hastening when the end to be desired requires time. The effort of those who are enlightened as the therapeutic law must ultimately, if slowly, illuminate the medical world (Hussey 1912).

7.1.2 Close

Close (1924) in his chapter on the *Repetition of Dose* argues:

It remains to speak of one more important matter connected with the general subject of Homoeopathic Posology - the repetition of the dose. The management of the remedy in regard to potency and dosage is almost as important as the selection of the remedy itself. The selection of the remedy can hardly be said to be finished until the potency and dosage have been decided upon.

These three factors, remedy, potency and dosage, are necessarily involved in the operation of prescribing. Not one of them is a matter of indifference and not one of them can be disregarded.

The first question which confronts us is whether to give one dose or repeated doses. The second question is, if we give one dose when shall we repeat it? Third, if we give repeated doses, how often shall we repeat the doses and when shall we stop dosing?

Many expert prescribers begin the treatment of practically all cases by giving a single dose of the indicated remedy and awaiting reaction. This is an almost ideal method - for expert prescribers. Of course we all expect to become expert prescribers and will therefore accept that as our ideal!

Hahnemann's usual teaching, the outcome of his long and rich experience, was to give a single dose and await its full action. The wisdom of this teaching has been amply confirmed since his day by many of his followers. The duration of action of a remedy which acts (and no other counts) varies, of course, with the nature and rate of progress of the disease. In a disease of such violence and rapid tendency toward death as cholera, for example, the action of the indicated remedy might be exhausted in five or ten minutes and another dose be required at the end of that time. In a slowly progressing chronic disease, like tuberculosis, the action of a dose of a curative remedy might continue for two or three months. Between these two extremes are all degrees of variation.

The only rule which can be laid down with safety is to repeat the dose only when improvement ceases. To allow a dose, or a remedy, to act as long as the improvement produced by it is sustained, is good practice; but to attempt to fix arbitrary limits to the action of medicine, as some have done, is contrary to experience.

Young practitioners and many old ones too, for that matter, give too many doses, repeat too frequently, change remedies too often. They give no time for reaction. they get doubtful, or hurried, or careless and presently they get "rattled" if the case is serious. Then it is "all up with them," until or unless they come to their senses and correct their mistakes. Sometimes such mistakes cannot be corrected and a patient pays the penalty with his life. It pays to be careful and "go slow" in the beginning; then there will not be so many mistakes to correct. We should examine our case carefully and systematically, select our first remedy and potency with care, give our first dose, if the single dose is decided upon and then watch results. If the remedy and dose are right there will be results. We need have no doubt on that score. The indicated remedy and potency, even in a single dose cannot be given without some result and the result must be good. Generally speaking, it may be taken for granted that if there is no perceptible result a reasonable time, depending upon the nature of the case, either the remedy or the potency was wrong.

One of the most difficult things is to learn to wait. three things are necessary; wisdom, courage and patience. "Strong doses" and frequent repetition will not avail if the remedy is not right.

In Par. 245 Hahnemann gives this general rule: "Perceptible and continued progress of improvement in an acute or chronic disease, is a condition which, as it lasts, invariably counterindicates the repetition of any medicine whatever, because the beneficial effect which the medicine continues to exert is rapidly approaching its perfection. Under these circumstances every new dose of medicine would disturb the process of recovery."

In the long note to Par. 246, however, which should be carefully studied, Hahnemann qualifies this statement and indicates the circumstances under which it is advisable to repeat the doses of the same remedy, using the action of *Sulphur* in chronic diseases as an illustration.

In Pars. 247 - 8, Hahnemann says: "These periods" (marked by the repetition of doses)" are always to be determined by the more or less acute course of the disease and by the nature of the remedy employed". the dose of the same medicine is to be repeated several times, if necessary, but only until recovery ensues, or until the remedy ceases to produce improvement; at that period the remainder of the disease, having suffered a change in its group of symptoms, requires another homoeopathic medicine." Study also Pars. 249 - 252.

The single dose of the indicated remedy, repeated whenever improvement ceases, as long as new or changed symptoms do not indicate a change of remedy, is adapted to all cases, but especially to chronic cases and to such acute cases as can be seen frequently and watched closely. The nature and progress of the disease will determine, under this rule, how often the dose is to be repeated. Cases may present themselves, however, which cannot be watched as closely as we would like. We may not be able to visit the patient frequently, nor remain with him long enough to observe the full period of remedial action. In such cases it is permissible and indeed necessary, to order a repetition of doses at stated intervals of one, two, or three hours, until improvement is felt or seen, or perhaps until our next visit. In such cases it is well to direct that the medicine be stopped as soon as the patient is better, giving some simple instruction to the nurse as to what constitutes a reliable sign of improvement, according to the nature of the case.

If a patient is so gravely ill as to require doses at intervals of less than one hour it is the physician's duty to remain with the patient and judge of his condition and progress for himself, unless he is absolutely sure of the remedy, or is in telephonic communication with the case.

Effect of the Remedy

The next point to be considered under the general subject of Homoeopathic Posology is: The Effect of the Remedy.

After we have selected what we believe to be the indicated remedy and administered it in proper potency and dosage, it is our duty to observe the patient carefully in order that we may correctly note and intelligently interpret the changes that occur; for upon these changes in the patient's condition, as revealed by the symptoms, depend our subsequent action in the further treatment of the case.

The first thing to be determined is whether the remedy has acted at all or not. If it has not acted, we have next to determine whether the failure to act is due to an error in the selection of the remedy, or to the selection of the wrong potency of the remedy. If, in carefully reviewing our symptom-record, we find the remedy rightly chosen, we change the potency to a higher or lower potency, as circumstances may require, after a reconsideration of the patient's degree of susceptibility.

In deciding the question whether the remedy has acted or not, we must be careful not to be misled by the opinions or prejudices of the patient or his attendants. Some patients, having all their interest and attention centered upon some particular symptom which they regard as all important, will assert that there has been no change; that they are no better, or even worse than they were before they took the remedy. These statements should be received with great caution and we should proceed to go over the symptom record item by item with care. We need not antagonize the patient by gruffly asserting that he must be mistaken, but may express our regret or sympathy and then quietly question him as to each particular symptom. We will frequently find that the patient has really improved in many important respects, although his pet symptom (often constipation) is as yet unchanged.

The action of a remedy is shown by changes in the symptoms of the patient. Upon the character of those changes depends our further course of action. A remedy shows its action, 1. by producing new symptoms; 2. by the disappearance of symptoms; 3. by the increase or aggravation of symptoms; 4. by the amelioration of symptoms; 5. by a change in the order and direction of symptoms (Close 1924).

7.1.3 Banerjee: The First Prescription

Banerjee (1984) in *The First Prescription* continues:

The next thing that should engage our attention after the prescription has been made and the potency fixed upon, is the question of regulation of dose. Whether to give only one single dose of the selected remedy and then wait until re-action sets in, or to give several doses in succession and stop when re-action is perceived to have begun. This is a matter that has to be decided by the sensitiveness of the patient's mind and physique. If the patient looks likely to have re-action from a single dose, there should be no repetition at all, as this may cause severe aggravation. But in cases where the patients are not sensitive enough, and as such there is likely to be delay in re-action, it is better to give a few repeated doses and then stop as soon as reaction is perceived to have commenced. In repeating doses like this, Hahnemann has advised in the sixth edition of his *Organon* that every succeeding dose should be of a slightly higher potency, and the method of increasing the potency in such cases has also been laid down there.

But how to ascertain that one single dose of a selected remedy is sufficient to excite re-action in one given case, and that in another some repeated doses are necessary?-If the patient is extremely nervous, if he is frightened easily, if he is pleased and displeased easily, or if he has ever before given indication of re-action on a very few doses of medicine, it is to be understood that he is a sensitive patient, and in that case, one single dose is enough and it should never be repeated, or, if after the use of the first dose there is some change perceived on the next day, there should be no repetition, and you should wait until the action of the dose given is exhausted. If however, on the contrary, the patient appears to be not easily impressionable and if he is not very weak, and as such, is likely to stand the re-action even if it be a bit severe, repeated doses may be given for a few days and then stopped when re-action has commenced. If again the patient's sufferings are not severe, the dose may be repeated until re-action begins. But in all other cases in which the patient is very weak, the potency to be used should be comparatively low and the repetition of the dose should also be carefully avoided. In fact, the whole condition of the patient should be carefully studied up and the question of repetition of dose dispassionately considered. The main thing that should be borne in mind is, that your object is to obtain a response from the patient to the medicine used, and if you gauge that one single dose is enough for this purpose, you must wait for a reasonable time and you must not repeat the dose until you perceive the response. If however, you think that several doses will be necessary, you may repeat until you get the response. You must remember that to give a single dose in a case where repeated doses are really necessary and to wait and wait, and to give repeated doses in a case where a single dose is sufficient to excite re-action, are equally bad. Because in the first case you lose time unnecessarily, while in the second you subject your patient to a lot of avoidable sufferings of a severe aggravation. You cannot therefore be over-cautious in this matter, and the fact remains that you must not repeat the dose when there is re-action, and that you must repeat the dose, even if it be at the rate of one dose daily, when there is delay in re-action, because all these repeated doses when given before the setting in of the re-action, will act like one single dose.

In acute cases, the action of a medicine is perceived in a few minutes (eg., in cholera etc.) or at the utmost in a few hours, but such is not the case in chronic cases. The first symptoms of the action of a medicine in a chronic case are hardly seen in less than 5 or 6 days, while in certain cases it may take even 3 or 4 weeks or more. In chronic cases, therefore, you have to wait patiently and observe the action of the medicine used, with care.

It has already been stated before, that the first prescription in a chronic case is a highly weighty business and that there should be no mistake in it, and I repeat the same thing again, as it is very very important. A correct first prescription in a chronic case really means half the cure for your patient and an immeasurable simplification of your work. But if unfortunately, there is a mistake in the first prescription, that is to say, if a wrong medicine has been given, we must learn the process of detecting it as also of taking remedial measures. This leads us to the following questions: (1) What should be the symptoms for indicating that the medicine used has been wrong? (2) How to remedy this? (3) How to understand that the medicine has been correct? (4) How to make sure that the potency also has been correct? (5) What should be the symptoms for indicating that the correct medicine has been used?

Before I undertake to explain the above problems, I should begin by saying that, like acute cases the treatment of chronic cases cannot possibly be carried on by examining the patient at the will of his guardian. In chronic treatment, the physician must have the privilege of making his examination of the patient whenever he considers it necessary, because the guardian of the patient or even the patient himself cannot understand as to when an examination of him is necessary. The physician only knows what developments he expects after the use of his medicine and what developments and aggravations he will hail with delight as symptoms of a process of cure and what he will view with alarm and try to remedy. It is therefore, that the physician will examine his patient whenever he considers it necessary, and unless there are facilities for this, there can be no chronic treatment.

Now, to the point. (1) and (2) If after the medicine used, there is a development of such symptoms as the patient has never experienced before in the whole course of his sufferings, it is to be understood that the selection has not been correct. It is a fact that in chronic cases patients are in the habit of having this and that occasionally, say a headache, an attack of dysentery, or fever etc; and if some such thing appears there as has never appeared before and if the patient is troubled with that, the evident conclusion should be that the prescription has not been correct. In such a case however, some antidote has to be used if the suffering is severe. If however, the suffering of the patient is not so severe, it is better to wait and allow the action of the wrong medicine to pass off completely, before a fresh prescription for the chronic disease is attempted. But, if this freshly selected medicine happens to be an antidote to the wrongly used medicine, then it should be given at once without any waiting for the passing off of its bad effects, as waiting in such a case would only be waste of time and unnecessary suffering to the patient.

I have explained the method of detecting the mistake, if any, in the first prescription as also of remedying it (i.e. questions 1 and 2 above), and I shall elucidate the remaining three questions (3, 4, and 5) in the next chapter.

Study of the effect of the first prescription

Let us now understand (3) how to make sure that the first prescription has been correct and that the potency used has also not been wrong. We have already understood that the appearance of new symptoms, such as have never troubled the patient before, will indicate that the first medicine has been wrong. Now, if exactly the opposite thing happens, that is to say, if only such symptoms as have troubled the patient before appear after the use of the medicine, it is to be understood that the medicine has been correct. But only the re-appearance of some of the old symptoms is not enough to indicate that it is the process of cure that has commenced. Something more is necessary, and it is this, that the old symptoms re-appear in the reverse order, that is to say, the last symptom in the patient will re-appear first and in this way all the old symptoms one after another and last of all the oldest symptom. If this is the order of the re-appearance of the old symptoms, then it should be recognised at once as the true process of cure, and as such the first medicine used should be considered to have been perfectly correct. Suppose, for example, it appears from the record of your case that the patient had malarial fever and that this was treated with quinine, and that after that he had dyspepsia, and suppose some Ayurvedic medicine suppressed that dyspepsia, and suppose simultaneously with the disappearance of the dyspepsia the patient had palpitation of the heart and vertigo etc., and last of all there came up dropsy and jaundice. Suppose, from this record you select a medicine according to the law of similarity and administer the first dose in the right potency. Now, what will happen if the medicine used has been correctly selected? The patient will be relieved first of all (but gradually) of his jaundice and dropsy, and his palpitation and vertigo will re-appear, and then these will pass off gradually, and then will re-appear the old dyspepsia, and then last of all will re-appear the old malarial fever. If this be the order of the re-appearance of the old symptoms-reverse order of their coming-under the use of your medicine, it is the process of cure. But if on the contrary, the old symptoms re-appear in a disorderly manner e.g., the malarial fever first, the palpitation then and last of all the dyspepsia, it is no process of cure. However, besides the process of cure being a re-appearance of the old symptoms in the reverse order of their coming, there are other indications also for judging the correctness of the medicine used, e.g., under the use of the correct medicine and in a process of cure which results from the use of the correct medicine, the process of re-appearance of the old symptoms is from within outward, from the more internal to the less internal organ, from the centre to the circumference, from the mind to the body, and from above downwards. This process is ever the process of cure and this invariably indicates that the right medicine has been used.

(4) But what is there to indicate that the right potency has been used? It is quite possible that in a given case you have used the

right medicine but not the right potency, and in such a case there will be no effect. It is therefore essentially necessary also to fix upon the right potency. The mere similarity of the symptoms of the drug with the totality of the symptoms of the case is not enough. The strength, that is to say, the potency of the drug must also be similar to the strength or the potency of the disease which you want to cure. That is to say that, the medicine must be so powerful (neither more nor less) as to be able to encounter the disease. This suggests that there is a "plane" in which the disease is, and your medicine also, must be fine and subtle enough to reach that "plane". Unless it is so, no cure can be expected. If however, you are quite sure that you have selected the right medicine for your patient and if there is no re-action yet in spite of a reasonable waiting, do not hasten to change the medicine at once, but consider carefully if the potency has to be changed, either for a higher or for a lower one. A change of medicine, just where only a change of potency is required on account of the correct potency having not been given in the first instance, creates quite a disaster at times. Want of re-action from the use of the correct medicine, in spite of a reasonable waiting should indicate that the correct potency has not perhaps been used.

(5) Now, what are we to expect on the use of the right medicine in the right potency? This is a difficult subject and let us discuss it in details.

The observation of the patient after the use of the first dose

Let us take for granted that the first prescription has been correct and that the prescribed medicine has been administered in the right potency. But what are we to expect now? When will the dose have to be repeated or a fresh selection made? How long are we to wait? Are there any indications for judging whether the patient will be cured? These are facts that will engage our attention now. But let me, in the mean time, tell you once again that, if repeated doses of the first medicine have been given as prescribed by Hahnemann in the sixth edition of the *Organon*, then the medicine must be stopped, directly re-action begins to appear, that is to say, there must be no more repetition of doses when there has been some change in the symptoms of the patient. And we must consider all the several doses that have been repeated to be as good as one single dose, because, though in number the doses have been so many, the effect is cumulative, and as such, it is the effect of one single dose in fact. There has been only one single stroke dealt to the life-force. For the life-force the doses that have produced no re-action, are no doses at all. The life-force did not feel them, and as such, they are all non-entities for it. This is why it is to be understood that in cases begun with repeated doses, all the doses repeated till before the appearance of re-action are to be considered as one single dose. However, when the re-action has appeared, that is to say, when there has been some change in the patient's symptoms, we must stop the medicine forthwith and watch the character and progress of the changes.

What are we to expect after the appearance of re-action on the use of the first dose? We are to expect some changes e.g.,- aggravation of disease symptoms or their amelioration, or their disappearance, or even a disorderly re-appearance of the old symptoms as distinct from their orderly re-appearance, which is always in the reverse order. Let us consider these different kinds of changes one by one.

In case of aggravation of the disease symptoms, we have to carefully analyze the aggravation. As for example, what is it that has been aggravated, and of what type and character is this aggravation? There may be an aggravation of the symptoms but the patient may yet feel better in his interior - in his mind. There may have been a rise in the temperature; the stools may have increased in number and even become worse in character, but yet, if the patient feels more at ease than before, it must be understood that the aggravation is a homoeopathic aggravation and that the patient is therefore improving. This aggravation is only an unmasking of that portion of the malady that was masked (suppressed), and is therefore, to the benefit of the patient, and you must not be unnerved at it. Then again, the patient may at times be unable to realise his own condition after the aggravation, that is to say, whether he is feeling better in the interior, and may not therefore tell you whether he is better or worse. And in such a case, you have to watch him out carefully and understand for yourself if he seems to be comparatively less morose and pulled down than before. If you find him like this, take it that it is homoeopathic aggravation, and there should therefore be no worrying over it. If however, instead of a homoeopathic aggravation (i,e. aggravation of the symptoms of the disease with an amelioration of the condition of the internal being of the patient), there is an aggravation of the disease symptoms as also of the internal (the mind) of the patient, it must be viewed with distrust, as, such an aggravation does not indicate the process of cure. In the case of a true homoeopathic aggravation, which indicates the process of cure, the patient must be better in the mind, in spite of the increase of his physical sufferings.

But why are we to accept a homoeopathic aggravation (aggravation of the physical symptoms of disease with an amelioration of the mental condition of the patient) as a favourable indication and the reverse of it as unfavourable? The fact is that the really curative medicine will begin its process of work from the centre to the circumference, and if it begins its work first in the centre, in the mind, the effect will be manifested at once in the mind, and the patient will therefore feel better mentally first. But if, on the contrary, the medicine only brings about some improvement in the external symptoms without bringing about relief in the mind, it only means that the medicine is not acting from the centre to the circumference, and as such it is no process of cure. The only process of cure, as has already been explained before, is from the centre to the circumference, from the more internal to the less internal, from above downwards and not otherwise.

Just here, I must make clear to you one very important fact. Before you use the first dose of your medicine in a chronic case, you must make sure that the patient has vitality enough to stand the homoeopathic aggravation that will follow. Because, unless there is sufficient strength in your patient to bear the sufferings of a temporary homoeopathic aggravation, he may altogether succumb under your medicine. This is a disaster that you must carefully avoid. (Banerjee1984a).

7.1.4 Banerjee: The Second Prescription

He then continues in his chapter on *The Second Prescription* Banerjee (1984b):

Let us now consider when the medicine prescribed at the first instance (first prescription) will have to be changed and the second prescription made.

If, after the amelioration obtained from the use of the first prescription, the original symptoms return, that is to say, if the original picture of the patient on which the first prescription was made, is presented again in the same form or in a milder form, it is to be understood that the potency used has not been high enough for effecting a total cure, and as such the disease force was only partially controlled and is showing itself up again. In such a case the same medicine will have to be repeated in a higher potency, so that the disease force may be completely controlled and eradicated and the life-force restored to its normal condition. But, if instead of the original picture, a new picture consisting of some new symptoms is presented, it is to be understood that the first prescription was not altogether correct. At times, it is the symptoms of the first medicine that appear, or in other words, the patient appears to be proving the remedy. In such cases, the first prescription has not only to be taken to have failed to cure the patient but has also to be taken to have done some positive mischief, by complicating the original picture with some drug symptoms. In such a case, one single group will have to be made of the whole array of symptoms now available, that is to say, the original picture of the patient plus the drug symptoms brought on by the erroneous selection will have to be considered as presenting one picture, and a fresh selection made correctly on that. If this second prescription is correctly made, it is sure that it will be quite a different medicine, that it will be by no means the medicine that was prescribed at the first instance.

In the above case, one thing should, however, be studied with care - namely, the condition of the "internal" of the patient - the condition of the patient's mind. If inspite of the appearance of some new symptoms the patient seems to be more at ease in the interior, then there should be no interference with a second medicine so long as this internal improvement of the patient lasts, merely on account of a few new symptoms having made their appearance. It may be that with some more waiting, the original symptoms will return and call for a higher potency of the same medicine, or it may be that this internal feeling of ease will gradually disappear and there will remain then the additional new symptoms only that had cropped up. In this last case there is no other alternative than to make a second prescription. Let me however, explain why I have advised waiting in case of new symptoms attended with an internal improvement of the patient. The fact is that these symptoms which the patient describes as "new", may not be really new. Perhaps they appeared in the course of the patient's disease or perhaps in his childhood, and it is possible that the patient did not either notice them or has forgotten them altogether. For this reason, whenever there is the slightest feeling of internal ease, it is all very wise to wait. In chronic treatment, waiting is a great thing. The slightest doubt or indecision should make you wait and watch. Now, in the present case, what are we to wait for? For a return of the symptoms on which the first prescription was made. If they do not return at all, and if the patient is also ceasing to feel the internal ease and improvement, there is no other help than to resort to a second prescription.

The stage for repeating the dose

It is necessary to know, as to when and on what definite indications the second dose has to be given. There are cases in which a hasty repetition of the dose, either due to the over-anxiety of the patient's guardian or due to want of patience on the part of the physician has caused serious mischief. Let us, therefore, bear in mind that, there should be no second dose unless it is called for by the indications of the case, because, it is not only that such a dose is unnecessary but also that it is positively mischievous. It must also be mentioned here that the occasion for a second dose, I am speaking of, may be there only when the first prescription has been correctly made and when as a result of that, the patient has made some response to the medicine. These advices must sound meaningless to those who care only for curing acute cases, as in acute cases there is no such all round response from the patient, but only a disappearance of symptoms. It is of course a fact, that there is perhaps not a single man who is not a chronic patient these days. But that does not necessarily mean that a chronic treatment will have to be made of every case that comes to you. Suppose, for example, here is an asthmatic coming to you for treatment. He complains "Sir, I have an awful dyspnœa and cough at about 2 or 3 in the morning. Pray, do something for me; but as I am unable to stay here for a week or so, you will have to cure me quickly." Now, suppose, you give him a few doses of Kali Bichrom. or Ars. or some such remedy as indicated by his symptoms, in the 30th potency, and the patient is relieved of his dyspnœa and other attendant symptoms in a week. But this is not chronic treatment. Or suppose, the above patient comes to you for a full course of chronic treatment, but if you treat him as above and quiet down his sufferings with low potencies like the 30th or 200th, it is no chronic treatment either, though the patient's is a good case for a course of chronic treatment, because by such potencies as 30th or 200th you only remove his symptoms and relieve him of his sufferings, without annihilating the possibility of similar sufferings in the future, and this is purely acute treatment-which is always therapeutic patchwork. Chronic treatment, on the other hand, is an annihilation of the miasmatic basis of all disease manifestations and it ensures immunity from all future diseases, whether in the shape of asthma or in any other shape. Therefore, for a physician who cares only for removing the particular disease manifestation, the second or third doses, or second or third prescriptions etc. are all unintelligible verbosity. The question of a second dose or third dose may only arise in the case of chronic treatment, and the course of such treatment is long enough. It takes time from one to five, six or seven years, or even more. Dr. Kent took 11 years to cure a patient who had chorea.

When however the patient does not want to undergo a course of chronic treatment though it may be necessary for a real cure of the man as a whole, high potencies should not be used. It is advisable to deal such cases with the 6th, 12th or the 30th at the utmost, because higher potencies might bring back the old symptoms at once and thereby necessitate a course of chronic treatment. Besides, it would only weaken the vital force unnecessarily; as the return of old symptoms, unless the case is treated to the end, means only a turmoil in the system, without any subsequent gain in strength on account of there being no final cure.

Now, after the use of the first dose of the first prescription, if it has been correctly made, there is bound to be a change in the symptoms of the patient. And during the course of this change, some of those symptoms on which the selection was made will be disappearing and re-appearing, while some of the others will be aggravated and some ameliorated. Thus, this period of change will be a period of disorder, in the sense that there will be nothing stationary. And so long as this condition of "change and turmoil" continues, that is to say, so long as the condition of the patient does not settle down into a definite state of quietness indicating that the action of the first dose has been exhausted, there should be no interference with a second dose. The changed condition of the patient would tempt the physician into repeating the medicine but this should never be done, because these changes only show that the medicine is acting, and therefore, there must be no interference so long as it acts, that is to say, so long as these changes continue. It is only when these changes, this appearance and disappearance of symptoms and their aggravation and amelioration have passed away, and when the condition of the patient has reached a stage of quietness, i.e., without any further changes, indicating that the medicine already given has almost ceased to act, that the question of a second dose should arise. It must be carefully remembered that any dose during the period of fleeting changes, after the first medicine, will spoil the whole case.

It is clear now, that after the first dose of the first prescription there will be some fleeting changes and after these there will be a condition of calmness, in which there will be no constant change of symptoms. This "calm" will indicate that the action of the medicine has been exhausted and that some medicine has to be given now. You will, therefore, have to watch carefully and see if any of the symptoms on which your first prescription was based is returning. If your first prescription was correct, and if it was allowed to act without any interference with any other medicine, then those symptoms must return. There is no doubt about that. Thus, a mere condition of calmness after a series of changes is not all you want for repeating the dose. For giving a second dose, the return of the symptoms on which you made your first prescription is necessary, and when these have returned, the second dose should be given at once without any further waiting. The return of these symptoms will show that the treatment so far has been perfectly correct-that the first prescription has been

Repetition of the Dose

perfectly homoeopathic and that it has been allowed to act long enough without any interference. It is however not possible to say how long it may take for the original symptoms, (on which the first prescription was made) to return. It may take one or two months and even a full year at times. Each individual case is its own rule in this matter and no other rule can be laid down. The time taken is however always in proportion to a large number of factors, e.g., the age, the vitality and the susceptibility of the patient, the chronicity of the case, the potency of the medicine used and so on.

It may be argued that the advice for waiting after the use of the first dose is intelligible enough, but what should be the course to be followed in cases, where there is no change even after a long waiting? This has already been explained to some extent, but let me say again that, in such cases, so that you may not have to wait too long after the first dose, you should repeat the dose every day or every alternate day slightly increasing the potency, as advised in the 6th edition of the *Organon*, and stop the dose as soon as some action of the medicine is perceived. This will avoid the risk of losing time unnecessarily, which may happen in case only one single dose of the medicine is used and in case when there is no re-action from that and yet you wait long enough. The repetition of the dose in increasingly higher potencies will accelerate the action, while stopping it simultaneously with the setting in of the re-action will not make all the several doses so many different units of action, but a single unit cumulated. In fact, the action obtained from such repeated doses is just like the action of one single dose, while there is no loss of time. If, however, there is no sign of re-action even after such repetition of doses, the mental condition of the patient should be studied at that stage, as it may be possible that there has been some improvement in the mind though it has not yet been reflected in the physical body. If there is some improvement in the mind, it is to be understood that the medicine has been acting, and in that case there should be no more doses and the action should be allowed to continue until the fleeting changes gradually appear and pass off and until there is a "calm" indicating the occasion for a second dose. If, however, from a study of the mental condition no improvement is perceived, it would become necessary to consider the correctness of the potency used, and you should then go higher up if the potency appears to have been too low.

It however happens at times, that after the fleeting changes that occur on the use of the first dose, there is a long interval and there is no prospect of a return of the symptoms on which the first prescription was made. This stage is a stage of no symptoms. There is no appearance and disappearance of symptoms and yet those symptoms on which the first prescription was made are altogether absent. Practically there are no symptoms, or very few symptoms at this stage. It may therefore lead you to repeat the dose but you must avoid such repetition at any cost. You are a true Homœopath and you must understand that you made your first prescription as justified by the symptoms. There has been re-action from your prescription too, but this re-action has ceased and a stage of no symptoms has come in. It must be that the re-action is still continuing, only that it is not being perceived on the outside. Possibly the medicine is acting in the furthest interior of the patient's being. Possibly it is now setting the disorders in the innermost corners right and has therefore no time to show its action on the surface, and possibly it will act on the surface only when it has finished correcting the interior. In such cases, you have, therefore, to wait. You must not repeat the dose and you must not try a new prescription. You must not repeat the dose, as an additional dose when the medicine already given is acting, will bring on a severe aggravation; while you cannot try a second prescription, as there are no symptoms to prescribe upon. You have, therefore, to wait in such cases, and if you wait and watch for some time, you will find that the symptoms on which you prescribed will re-appear.

Whenever you are tempted to repeat the dose or to re-prescribe in such cases, you should weigh the situation and argue that a number of symptoms are constantly coming and going and there is nothing certain - no totality of symptoms to prescribe upon, and therefore, there should be no prescription. Similarly, when there is a stage of no symptoms, there can be no prescription too, because, as a Homœpath, you cannot prescribe without having a totality of symptoms to prescribe upon. It is this very sound logic that should keep you from repeating the dose and from prescribing afresh during the stage of fleeting changes that comes after the first prescription as also during the stage of no symptoms that follows the stage of fleeting changes. This logic should therefore make you wait and watch, and there is no doubt that, the condition - the basis of your first prescription will soon return and offer you a case for a second dose of the same medicine either in the same or in a higher potency.

After the use of the second dose there will be a change again and perhaps a re-appearance of the symptoms on which you prescribed, just as after the use of the first dose. This may repeat several times, and at every repetition of dose you should try to use a higher potency i.e., as far as permitted by the gradual gain in vitality by the patient. And gradually there will re-appear the old symptoms that had disappeared and these will then gradually disappear of themselves indicating that a total cure has been effected. If however, you watch very carefully, you will find one very marvellous fact at all the several re-appearances of the symptoms on which the prescription was based, and it is this the patient will be ever feeling greater and greater ease and relief in his mind inspite of all the physical symptoms. This is a fact that will furnish you an unmistakable evidence of the correctness of your selection. How very beautiful! Just imagine, the patient has all the symptoms for which you prescribed and perhaps in an aggravated form, and yet he is feeling better in the mind! (Banerjee 1984b).

7.1.5 Close Again

Stuart Close (1924) in *Posology and Repetition* argues:

Homoeopathic Posology: By posology (from the Greek, posos, how much) we mean the science or doctrine of dosage.

Repetition of Doses - It remains to speak of one more important matter connected with the general subject of Homoeopathic Posology - the repetition of the dose. The management of the remedy in regard to potency and dosage is almost as important as the selection of the remedy itself. The selection of the remedy can hardly be said to be finished until the potency and dosage have been decided upon. These three factors, remedy, potency and dosage, are necessarily involved in the operation of prescribing. Not one of them is a matter of indifference and not one of them can be disregarded.

The first question which confronts us is whether to give one dose or repeated doses. The second question is, if we give one dose when shall we repeat it? Third, if we give repeated doses, how often shall we repeat the doses and when shall we stop dosing?

Many expert prescribers begin the treatment of practically all cases by giving a single dose of the indicated remedy and awaiting reaction. This is an almost ideal method-for expert prescribers. Of course we all expect to become expert prescribers and will therefore accept that as our ideal!

Hahnemann's usual teaching, the outcome of his long and rich experience, was to give a single dose and await its full action. The wisdom of this teaching has been amply confirmed since his day by many of his followers. The duration of action of a remedy which acts (and no other counts) varies, of course, with the nature and rate of progress of the disease. In a disease of such violence and rapid tendency toward death as cholera, for example, the action of the indicated remedy might be exhausted in five or ten minutes and another dose be required at the end of that time. In a slowly progressing chronic disease, like tuberculosis, the action of a dose of a curative remedy might continue for two or three months. Between these two extremes are all degrees of variation.

The only rule which can be laid down with safety is to repeat the dose only when improvement ceases. To allow a dose, or a remedy, to act as long as the improvement produced by it is sustained, is good practice; but to attempt to fix arbitrary limits to the action of medicine, as some have done, is contrary to experience.

Young practitioners and many old ones too, for that matter, give too many doses, repeat too frequently, change remedies too often. They give no time for reaction. They get doubtful, or hurried, or careless and presently they get "rattled" if the case is serious. Then it is "all up with them," until or unless they come to their senses and correct their mistakes. Sometimes such mistakes cannot be corrected and a patient pays the penalty with his life. It pays to be careful and "go slow" in the beginning; then there will not be so many mistakes to correct. We should examine our case carefully and systematically, select our first remedy and potency with care, give our first dose, if the single dose is decided upon and then watch results. If the remedy and dose are right there will be results. We need have no doubt on that score. The indicated remedy and potency, even in a single dose cannot be given without some result and the result must be good. Generally speaking, it may be taken for granted that if there is no perceptible result after a reasonable time, depending upon the nature of the case, either the remedy or the potency was wrong.

One of the most difficult things is to learn to wait. Three things are necessary; wisdom, courage and patience. "Strong doses" and frequent repetition will not avail if the remedy is not right.

In Par. 245 Hahnemann gives this general rule: "Perceptible and continued progress of improvement in an acute or chronic disease, is a condition which, as long as it lasts, invariably counter-indicates the repetition of any medicine whatever, because the beneficial effect which the medicine continues to exert is rapidly approaching its perfection. Under these circumstances every new dose of medicine would disturb the process of recovery."

In the long note to Par. 246, however, which should be carefully studied, Hahnemann qualifies this statement and indicates the circumstances under which it is advisable to repeat the doses of the same remedy, using the action of Sulphur in chronic diseases as an illustration.

In Pars. 247-8, Hahnemann says: "These periods" (marked by the repetition of doses) "are always to be determined by the more or less acute course of the disease and by the nature of the remedy employed. The dose of the same medicine is to be repeated several times, if necessary, but only until recovery ensues, or until the remedy ceases to produce improvement; at that period the remainder of the disease, having suffered a change in its group of symptoms, requires another homoeopathic medicine." Study also Pars. 249-252.

The single dose of the indicated remedy, repeated whenever improvement ceases, as long as new or changed symptoms do not indicate a change of remedy, is adapted to all cases, but especially to chronic cases and to such acute cases as can be seen frequently and watched closely. The nature and progress of the disease will determine, under this rule, how often the dose is to be repeated. Cases may present themselves, however, which cannot be watched as closely as we would like. We may not be able to visit the patient frequently, nor remain with him long enough to observe the full period of remedial action. In such cases it is permissible and indeed necessary, to order a repetition of doses at stated intervals of one, two, or three hours, until improvement is felt or seen, or perhaps until our next visit. In such cases it is well to direct that the medicine be stopped as soon as the patient is better, giving some simple instruction to the nurse as to what constitutes a reliable sign of improvement, according to the nature of the case.

If a patient is so gravely ill as to require doses at intervals of less than one hour it is the physician's duty to remain with the patient and judge of his condition and progress for himself, unless he is absolutely sure of the remedy, or is in telephonic communication with the case.

Effect of the Remedy: The next point to be considered under the general subject of Homoeopathic Posology is: The Effect of the

Remedy.

After we have selected what we believe to be the indicated remedy and administered it in proper potency and dosage, it is our duty to observe the patient carefully in order that we may correctly note and intelligently interpret the changes that occur; for upon these changes in the patient's condition, as revealed by the symptoms, depend our subsequent action in the further treatment of the case.

The first thing to be determined is whether the remedy has acted at all or not. If it has not acted, we have next to determine whether the failure to act is due to an error in the selection of the remedy, or to the selection of the wrong potency of the remedy. If, in carefully reviewing our symptom-record, we find the remedy rightly chosen, we change the potency to a higher or lower potency, as circumstances may require, after a reconsideration of the patient's degree of susceptibility.

In deciding the question whether the remedy has acted or not, we must be careful not to be misled by the opinions or prejudices of the patient or his attendants. Some patients, having all their interest and attention centered upon some particular symptom which they regard as all-important, will assert that there has been no change; that they are no better, or even worse than they were before they took the remedy. These statements should be received with great caution and we should proceed to go over the symptom-record item by item with care. We need not antagonize the patient by gruffly asserting that he must be mistaken, but may express our regret or sympathy and then quietly question him as to each particular symptom. We will frequently find that the patient has really improved in many important respects, although his pet symptom (often constipation) is as yet unchanged.

The action of a remedy is shown by changes in the symptoms of the patient. Upon the character of those changes depends our further course of action. A remedy shows its action, 1. by producing new symptoms; 2. by the disappearance of symptoms; 3. by the increase or aggravation of symptoms; 4. by the amelioration of symptoms; 5. by a change in the order and direction of symptoms.

1. An improperly chosen remedy may change the condition of an oversensitive patient by producing new symptoms not related to the disease and detrimental to his welfare. These are pathogenetic symptoms. Their appearance indicates that the remedy is not curing the patient, but merely making a proving. Discontinuance and an antidote is demanded.

2. A correctly chosen remedy given in too low or sometimes too high a potency, or in too many doses, may cause an aggravation of the existing symptoms so severe as to endanger the life of the patient; especially if the patient be a child or a sensitive person and if a vital organ, like the brain or lungs be affected. Belladonna in the third or sixth potency, given in too frequent doses in a case of meningitis, for example, may cause death from overaction; whereas the thirtieth or two hundredth potency given in a single dose, or in doses repeated only until some change of symptoms is noticed, will speedily cure. Phosphorus 3rd or 6th in pneumonia under similar circumstances may rapidly cause death. The low potencies of deeply acting medicines are dangerous in such cases in proportion to their similarity to the symptoms.

The more accurate the selection of the medicine, the greater must be the care exercised not to injure the patient by prescribing potencies too low and doses too numerous. Medication should be stopped on the first appearance of such aggravations. An antidote should be administered if they do not speedily diminish. The careless prescriber rarely recognizes such aggravations. When he notices the symptoms he usually attributes them to the natural course of the disease or calls it a "complication."

3. A slight aggravation or intensification of the symptoms, appearing quickly after giving the remedy and soon passing away is a good sign. It calls for a suspension of medication until the after-following improvement ceases or the symptoms change again. It is the first and best evidence of the curative action of a well chosen remedy.

4. A prolonged aggravation without amelioration and with progressive decline of the patient is sometimes seen in chronic, deep seated disease as a result of the over-action of a deeply acting anti-psoric or anti-syphilitic medicine, given in too high a potency in the beginning of treatment. If the potency is too high its action may be too deep and far-reaching, and the reaction too great for the weakened vital power to carry on. Such remedies as *Sulphur, Calcarea, Mercury, Arsenic* and *Phosphorus*, given in the 50 M. or C.M., potencies, have sometimes hastened tubercular or tertiary syphilitic cases into the grave. In beginning treatment of suspicious or possibly incurable cases it is better to use medium potencies, like the 30th or 200th and go higher gradually, if necessary, as treatment progresses and the patient improves.

Very high potencies of the closely similar remedy are merciless searchers-out of hidden things. They will sometimes bring to light a veritable avalanche of symptoms which overwhelms the weakened patient. The disease has gone too far for such radical probing. If the disease has not gone so far, a long and severe aggravation may fortunately be followed by slow improvement. That patient was on the "borderland," with the beginning of serious destructive change in some vital organ.

In these homoeopathic reactions and aggravations we distinguish between changes occurring in vital organs and changes in superficial tissues and non-vital organs. When old skin eruptions reappear, old ulcers break out again, old fistulæ re-open, old discharges flow again, swollen tubercular glands become inflamed, break down and suppurate away; old joint pains return; the patient's heart, lung, kidney, liver, spleen or brain symptoms in the meantime improving; then we know that both remedy and dose were right and a true cure is in progress. But if we find superficial symptoms disappearing and vital organs showing signs of advancing disease, we know we have failed.

The direction of cure is from within outward, from above downward and in the reverse order of the appearance of the symptoms. By this test we may always know whether we are curing or only palliating a disease. The last appearing symptoms of a disease should be the first to disappear under the action of a curative remedy.

In sub-acute and chronic diseases it is not unusual for preceding groups of symptoms to successively reappear as the later symptoms subside and cure progresses. This orderly change of symptoms should never be interfered with by repetition of doses nor change of remedy, so long as it continues. When improvement ceases or old symptoms reappear and remain without change it is time to repeat the dose.

5. The change following the administration of a remedy may be a quick, short amelioration followed by a relapse to the original or a worse condition. This may be because the remedy was only partly similar, or insufficient as to dosage; but where this occurrence is observed several times in succession and lasting improvement does not follow carefully selected remedies, it means that the case is incurable. There is not vitality enough to sustain a curative reaction, and dissolution is imminent.

6. In functional diseases, or in the beginning of acute organic diseases, accompanied perhaps by severe pain, the administration of the appropriate dose of the indicated remedy may be followed by rapid disappearance of symptoms without any aggravation. This is a cure of the most satisfactory kind, pleasing alike to physician and patient. Remedy and potency were both exactly right.

The Law of Dosage: Summing up the matter, it appears that the law of dosage is contained in the law of similars, or the law of equivalents, both of which expressions are merely para-phrases of the law of Mutual Action, otherwise known as Newton's third law of motion.

The law might be stated thus: The curative dose, like the remedy, must be similar in quantity and quality to the dose of the morbific agent which caused the disease.

I was taught, for example, that "low potencies acted best in acute diseases." I accepted that generalization and acted upon it for some time before I discovered that it was altogether too broad, if not entirely false. It was not long before I witnessed a cure of an acute disease by a two hundredth potency so rapid and brilliant that I was encouraged to put it to the test myself. I succeeded in a number of cases and then I failed in a certain case. When I reflected upon the exception and sought for a reason why the high potency had acted in ten similar cases and failed in one, I found it in the grosser type of the individual and his lower degree of susceptibility, as well as in the lower grade of his disease process. He required a grosser, more material, lower form of a remedy to cure him.

I was taught also that infants and aged persons, being of low vitality and feeble reactive powers, required low potencies for their cure. Again I found that the generalization was altogether too broad; for I have cured the most desperate cases of croup, diphtheria, cholera infantum, etc., with a few doses of a high potency after they have been given up to die by those who had been prescribing tinctures and low potencies without avail; and I have seen as brilliant curative effects of high potencies in the aged as in the young, when both the remedy and the potency were indicated. Again we must individualize. Low potencies will not cure all acute diseases, all infants, nor all aged persons. Nor will high potencies cure all forms of disease in all persons. All potencies are required for the cure of disease, and any potency may be required in any given case (Close 1934).

The collective insight of Hussey, Close, Banerjee and others still offer much for us with the challenges we face prescribing in the 21st century. While written long ago these represent the conservative foundational directives and principles from which we can operate effectively still.

Chapter 8 | The Rich Landscape of Posology

In this chapter you will:
1. Grasp the similarities and difference in approaches
2. Identify who advocated these approaches
3. Learn the literature that underpins the approaches

Chapter 8

The Rich Landscape of Posology

It is best to begin with some context.

8.1 Hahnemann's Timeline in the development and use of the 50 millesimal potencies

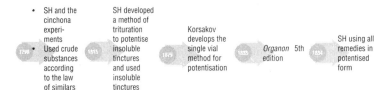

- SH and the cinchona experiments
- Used crude substances according to the law of similars

SH developed a method of trituration to potentise insoluble tinctures and used insoluble tinctures

Korsakov develops the single vial method for potentisation

Organon 5th edition

SH using all remedies in potentised form

Timeline of Hahnemann's development and use of the 50 millesimal potencies

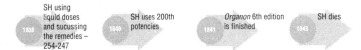

SH using liquid doses and sucussing the remedies – 254-247

SH uses 200th potencies

Organon 6th edition is finished

SH dies

Hahnemann develops and uses Q (LM) potencies from 1837-1843

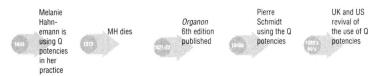

Melanie Hahnemann is using Q potencies in her practice

MH dies

Organon 6th edition published

Pierre Schmidt using the Q potencies

UK and US revival of the use of Q potencies

Post Hahnemann

8.2 Critical Thinking

Homeopathy is full of assertions. 'Never begin a case with *Lycopodium* 200'. It just lends itself to the one liner. The pithy aphorism. That's part of its tradition. And its charm. But can charm and soundbites be the basis for a body of knowledge, for a science?

'Never on your life give a remedy when the previous one is still working. It's bad it's wrong. It's criminal negligence! The homeopathic police will come along and lock you up,' said one of my lecturers. 'The finest curative action I ever observed was begun sixty days after the administration of the single dose' says Kent in *Lesser Writings*. 'The suppressed case always goes bad,' says Stuart Close.

These are some of the quotes I remember when I was studying homeopathy. They came from my teachers and the books. It was clear and unequivocal. They convinced me that the minimum dose concept meant just that. The minimum dose, (one dose) and wait. Repeat when the symptoms have returned. That was then. I knew it to be so.

What was more concerning however is when I found myself as lecturer to a group of undergraduate students saying something like, 'just wait, never prescribe a medicine when the action of the previous one is still acting. Just don't do it!' It is a concern to me that I was passing on 'knowledge' when it was neither founded on empiricism, on any form of rationalism, but heavily reliant on rhetoric, opinion and my techniques of public speaking (which are not too bad).

Critical evaluation of the literature on posology

While Kent often gets a bad rap these days, and is reputed to have said all sorts of things, it seems that it is from him where the beginnings of this 'knowledge' began in relationship to repetition of the dose (Treuherz 1984).

> The third great mistake which the homeopathic physician cannot too carefully avoid in the treatment of chronic diseases, is too hasty repetition of the dose. The three precautions of the master found in the *'Chronic Diseases'* should be printed and posted in every physician's office and committed to memory (Kent 1888).

> In chronic skin diseases you need not expect any change inside of two weeks, and sometimes you will have to wait two, three, or six months, so in these cases I administer a single dose, and it may be a month or two before I repeat. Some of the best cures I have ever made have been in cases where I have repeated not oftener than once in two or three months. Never repeat when the symptoms show signs of amelioration (Morgan 1895).

Vithoulkas

Kentian philosophy influenced generations of homeopaths. The most Kentian of them all, Vithoulkas trained and influenced most homeopaths from the 1970 and 80s, especially American and English teachers. He spread the same message as concrete knowledge.

He advocated a strong insistence to continue Hahnemann's old methods (what in fact was the 4th edition of *Chronic Diseases* and *Organon of Medicine*) of single dose and of dry pills. Moreover, there was a heavy emphasis on the use of centesimal potencies in Kent's sequencing 30, 200, M, 10M,

50M, CM. But actually Hahnemann often went down the potency scales as disease improved. However for Kent, anything else (repeated dose) in chronic disease was condemned a danger and carried with it the potential to mess up the case. Or worse, suppress, spoil or do irreparable damage to the case. A culture of fear, hesitancy and nervousness in prescribing has pervaded the profession ever since and still infects our classrooms. In addition, and often forgotten, is the audience that Kent and Close were lecturing to when they admonished their students. They lectured to allopathic physicians and not the Deepak Chopra, Louise Hay versed homeopathic students of today.

What Hahnemann Actually Said

There is always a problem in reverting back to the words of the master to justify a personally held belief. Homeopaths do it all the time. When it suits them that is. But this constant referencing back to Hahnemann to justify beliefs related to repetition of the dose has been so patchy, so selective and unrigourous. To my mind, the following passages are very important in creating clarity.

> Nevertheless the incredible variety among patients as to their irritability, their age, their spiritual and bodily development, their vital power and especially as to the nature of their disease, necessitates a great variety in their treatment, and also in the administration to them of the doses of medicine.
>
> For their diseases may be of various kinds: either a natural and simple one but lately arisen, or it may be a natural and simple one but an old case, or it may be a complicated one (a combination of several miasmata), or again what is the most frequent and worse

case, it may have been spoiled by a perverse medical treatment, and loaded down with medicinal disease.

Experience has shown me, as it has no doubt also shown to most of my followers, that it is most useful in diseases of any magnitude...to give the homoeopathic pellet or pellets only in solution, and this solution in divided doses.

...in chronic diseases I have found it best to give a dose (e.g.., a spoonful) of a solution of the suitable medicine at least every two days, more usually every day.

...But in taking one and the same medicine repeatedly (which is indispensable to secure the cure of serious chronic disease), if the dose is in every case varied and modified only a little in its degree of dynamisation, then the vital force of the patient will calmly, and as it were willingly receive the same medicine in succession with the best results, every time increasing the wellbeing of the patient.

This slight change in the degree of dynamisation is even effected, if the bottle which contains the solution of one or more pellets is merely shaken five or six times, every time before taking it.

...if the medicine continues useful, he will take one or two pellets of the same medicine in a lower potency (e.g., if before he had used the thirtieth dilution, he will now take one or two pellets of the twenty-fourth)

On any day when the remedy has produced too strong an action, the dose should be omitted for a day. If the symptoms of the disease alone appear, but are considerably aggravated even during the same moderate use of the medicine, then the time has come to break off in the use of the medicine for one or two weeks, and await a considerable improvement (Hahnemann 1986 p155-7).

It is also mentioned in Hahnemann's footnote that in acute diseases give spoonfuls of the dilution every ½ hour or hour or 2 hours depending on the need. Hahnemann then talks in some detail about rubbing the same medicine (as taken orally) onto healthy skin free from ailments to speed up the cure of chronic disease. First one un-affected limb (region) then another, alternating the region where the solution is rubbed in.

> ...but during the last years, since I have been giving every dose of the medicine in an incorruptible solution, divided over fifteen, twenty or thirty days and even more, no potentising in an attenuating vial is found too strong, and I again use ten strokes with each. So I herewith take back what I wrote on this subject three years ago in the first volume of this book on page 149.

He takes it back! He retracted what he wrote on the minimum dose in the 1st, 2nd, 3rd and 4th edition of *Chronic Diseases*. How therefore could Kent assert what he asserted about pills and waiting? He obviously didn't read the *Chronic Diseases* as he claimed. The mist between truth, belief and knowledge is very thick here!

A critical evaluation of the 5th and 6th editions of the *Organon of Medicine* also casts the same doubt on the legitimacy of this 'knowledge' as asserted by Kent and neo-Kentians. In Kent's defense, he never saw the 6th edition, Kent read the 4th edition, but that's no excuse for anyone else. In writing about the single dose, or repetition in chronic diseases, Hahnemann makes assertions in the 5th edition which he clearly changes and takes back in the 6th edition from new experience:

> ...Every perceptibly progressive and strikingly increasing amelioration in a transient (acute) or persistent (chronic) disease, is a condition which, as long as it lasts, completely precludes every

repetition of the administration of any medicine whatsoever, because all the good the medicine taken continues to effect is new hastening towards its completion. Every new dose of any medicine whatsoever, even of the one last administered, that has hitherto shown itself to be salutary, would in this case disturb the work of amelioration… (Hahnemann 1921 aphorism 245).

This aphorism is totally omitted in the 6th Edition.

On the other hand, the slowly progressive amelioration consequent on a very minute dose, whose selection has been accurately homeopathic, when it has met with no hindrance to the duration of its action, sometimes accomplishes all the good the remedy in question is capable from its nature of performing in a given case, in periods of forty, fifty or a hundred days. This is, however, but rarely the case; and besides, it must be a matter of great importance to the physician as well as to the patient that were it possible, this period should be diminished to one- half, one-quarter, and even still less, so that a much more rapid cure might be obtained. And this may be very happily affected, as recent and oft-repeated observations have shown, under three conditions: firstly, if the medicine selected with the utmost care was perfectly homeopathic; secondly, if it was given in the minutest dose, so as to produce the least possible excitation of the vital force, and yet sufficient to effect the necessary change in it; and thirdly, if this minutest yet powerful dose of the best selected medicine *be repeated at suitable intervals** which experience shall have pronounced to be the best adapted for accelerating the cure to the utmost extent, yet without the vital force, which it is sought to influence to the production of a similar medicinal disease, being able to feel itself excited and roused to adverse reactions" 5th ed 246.

Aphorism 246 is re-written in the 6th Edition:

Every perceptibly progressive and strikingly increasing amelioration during treatment is a condition which, as long as it lasts, completely precludes every repetition of the administration of any medicine whatsoever, because all the good the medicine taken continues to effect is now hastening towards its completion. This is not infrequently the cause in acute diseases, but in more chronic diseases, on the other hand, a single dose of an appropriately selected homeopathic remedy will at times complete even with but slowly progressive improvement and give the help which such a remedy in such a case can accomplish naturally within 40, 50, 60, 100 days.

This is, however, but rarely the case; and besides, it must be a matter of great importance to the physician as well as to the patient that were it possible, this period should be diminished to one-half, one-quarter, and even still less, so that a much more rapid cure might be obtained. And this may be very happily affected, as recent and oft-repeated observations have taught me under the following conditions: firstly, if the medicine selected with the utmost care was perfectly homoeopathic; secondly, if it is highly potentised, dissolved in water and given in proper small dose that experience has taught as the most suitable in definite intervals for the quickest accomplishment of the cure but with the precaution, *that the degree of every dose deviate somewhat from the preceding and following* in order that the vital principle which is to be altered to a similar medicinal disease be not aroused to untoward reactions and revolt as is always the case with unmodified and especially rapidly repeated doses.

Foot note; "What I said in the fifth edition of the *Organon*, in a long footnote to this paragraph in order to prevent these undesirable reactions of the vital energy, was all that experience I had justified. But during that last four or five years, however, all these difficulties are wholly solved by my new altered but perfected method. The same carefully selected medicine may now be given daily and for months, if necessary in this way namely, after the lower degree of potency has been used for one or two weeks in the treatment of a chronic disease, advance is made in the same way to the higher degrees, beginning according to the new dynamisation method, taught herewith with the use of the lowest degrees."

But if the succeeding dose is changed slightly every time, namely potentised somewhat higher (pp. 269 - 270) then the vital principle may be altered without difficulty by the same medicine (the sensation of natural disease diminishing) and thus the cure brought nearer. (Aphorism 247 Hahnemann 1921).

Aphorism 248 is re-written in the 6th Edition:

For this purpose, we potentise anew the medicinal solution (with perhaps 8, 10, 12 succussions) from which we give the patient one or (increasingly) several teaspoonful doses, in long lasting diseases daily or every second day, in acute diseases every two to six hours and in very urgent cases every hour or oftener. Thus in chronic diseases, every correctly chosen homeopathic medicine, even those whose action is of long duration, may be repeated daily for months with ever increasing success. If the solution is used up (in seven to fifteen days) it is necessary to add to the next solution of the same medicine if still indicated one or (though rarely) several pellets of a higher potency with which we continue so long as the patient experiences continued improvement without encountering one or another complaint that he never had before in his life.

For if this happens, if the balance of the disease appears in a group of altered symptoms then another, one more homoeopathically related medicine must be chosen in place of the last and administered in the same repeated doses, mindful, however, of modifying the solution of every dose with thorough vigorous succussions, thus changing its degree of potency and increasing it somewhat. On the other hand, should there appear during almost daily repetition of the well indicated homeopathic remedy, towards the end of the treatment of a chronic disease, so-called (& 161) homeopathic aggravations by which the balance of the morbid symptoms seem to again increase somewhat (the medicinal disease, similar to the original, now alone persistently manifests itself). The doses in that case must then be reduced still further and repeated in longer intervals and possibly stopped several days, in order to see if the convalescence need no further medicinal aid.

The apparent symptoms (Schein - Symptom) caused by the excess of the homeopathic medicine will soon disappear and leave undisturbed health in its wake. If only a small vial say a dram of dilute alcohol is used in the treatment, in which is contained and dissolved through succussion one globule of the medicine which is to be used by olfaction every two, three or four days, this also must be thoroughly succussed eight to ten times before each olfaction (Aphorism 248 6th ed. Hahnemann 1921).

It is perplexing that these homeopathic authorities asserted what they did in relation to repetition of the dose when Hahnemann, who they claim to have read and follow clearly, said and did something different. We have to assume that this 'knowledge' was based on their own experience, and the rhetoric of their masters, coaches and teachers. It certainly wasn't based on any homeopathic authority or precedent.

Application of *critical thinking* and evaluation shows there are faulty arguments, inductive generalizations, all sorts of assertions lacking rudimentary evidence other than analogy, and claims of truth based on flimsy philosophical systems. Kent claimed to have read Hahnemann's *Chronic Diseases*, but Hahnemann clearly wrote something in 1833 that is fundamentally different to Kent's assertions fifty years later regarding instructions on dosage. It is often pitched as *a priori* knowledge, but is at best a straight up myth. The reality is that Mathur does this. Sankaran does that. In seminars over the years, Sherr (Lecture Malvern 2003) gives two single doses of a centesimal a couple of hours apart. Scholten gives one dose of 1M and waits (Lecture Sydney 2001). My experience has led me to conclude like Bernoville in Sankaran's article (P Sankaran 1996), that, "As a rule we must stop repeating as soon as we have effect from the medicine applied." There can be no doubt that I have had very pleasing results from my early practice by applying the knowledge I had from my teachers via Kent. But I also experienced many poor results, and times when my prescriptions clearly underwhelmed my patient; results that then improved when I finally read articles like Sankaran's, actually read *Chronic Diseases* and the *Organon*, and started to challenge and analyse the beliefs I had about my practice.

Knowledge is not about yelling louder. That is rhetoric. It is not about name dropping. That creates sacred cows. Rhetoric is generally described as the art of persuasion through language. Rhetoric can be described as a persuasive way in which one relates a theme or idea in an effort to convince. It is often used in a dismissive sense, when someone wants to denigrate certain verbal reasoning as spurious. The term "sacred cow" is used for a person, institution, idea or ideology that is immune from criticism or opposition. It stems from the Hindu belief that the cow is sacred and holds an honoured place in society. The cow should not be moved, touched, harmed or interfered with in any way, no matter what. Knowledge comes from reading and experience. My advice is get both. My beliefs and the impact on my practice have been dramatically altered over the years from this critical evaluation and reflection. I genuinely thought I would harm, suppress and do damage to people with radical repetition ideas. But before I was less effective, now I am more effective. By using the 6th edition of the *Organon*, and the 5th when using centesimal potencies, the impact on my clients is that they take their medicine in a similar way to how they have taken their orthodox medicine previously – daily. It is less weird to them. My practice has changed. I see fewer patients who have seen a homeopath before. I see more conventional medicine rejects to whom homeopathy is new. The impact on them and me is that there is flexibility – I can dilute the dose, make it hourly daily, weekly, diluted in two litres of water if I wish. They get it. Moreover the biggest impact has been that our communication is better. There is a further impact - my clients are more involved in their treatment. They become a part of it. And take responsibility for it. We do it together as opposed to the Victorian doctor patient relationship of Kent. It serves to acknowledge that we are in this relationship together.

The impact has also been felt by my students who are less fearful and more confident in their prescribing especially in the early years of their practice. This is crucial. Moreover they do not see this area as a belief rather than concrete knowledge. We name it as such. For me, there can be no other conclusion that one of the great myths and sacred cows in homeopathic medicine has been the knowledge of minimum dose, second prescription, watch and wait technique. Previously I thought it was knowledge, now I see it as belief. This is not to say it's wrong. It still can be very useful and get results. But we should call it what it is. What has underpinned our 'knowledge' about this area has been experience and rhetoric, not rationality nor homeopathic authority. Most classical homeopaths perceive the ultimate homeopathic authority as Hahnemann. Yet Hahnemann never said or did what they say he said or did.

Learning from Authors who Have Read the Literature

It was only reading this article, *Repetition of the Dose*, from P Sankaran that made me question posology to such an extent:

> The repetition of doses: In homoeopathic practice, the selection of the proper remedy is probably the most essential thing, but after the remedy has been selected and administered in the proper potency, the homoeopathic physician should be able to watch out for, understand and interpret the remedy reaction and should know the proper "period for repeating the dose". This is considered so important that masters like Kent warn us that a case can be completely spoiled by improper repetition of the dose.

> Repetition in acute cases: In homoeopathic practice, in acute cases, the frequent repetition of doses, even of high potencies, seems to be generally and universally approved. Borland, for example, used to give in cases of pneumonia 1M or 10M every 2

hours. It is believed that in acute disease the pace of the disease is such that the effect of the doses is quickly exhausted.

It must however be mentioned that there were masters like Boger who were prescribing single doses even in acute cases. Dr. Boger mentions, for example, that he had never given more than one dose of the remedy in the hundreds of cases of typhoid that he had treated. But such prescribers are exceptional. I quote here some of my experiences in acute cases.

In the beginning, even in acute diseases I was taught not to repeat the dose until and unless the action of the previous dose had been completely exhausted. I was instructed for instance, that in a case of fever if the maximum temperature was 104°F on the day I prescribed, I should never repeat the remedy even if the patient continued to have fever until and unless the temperature went up to 104°F again. Even if the patient had continued or intermittent fever for a month, if the subsequent highest level of temperature after the dose of medicine was less than the original level, the remedy was not to be repeated because probably the previous dose was still acting. In the initial stages, I obeyed this teaching implicitly like Casabianca and possibly I lost many patients. But, gradually, I made one observation. In acute cases, I used to give my patients a number of doses but I used to instruct them strictly that the moment there was any evidence of improvement, e.g. in a case of fever as soon as the temperature started coming down, the doses were to be immediately discontinued. Some patients followed my advice to the letter but others did not. The latter who ignored my instructions and repeated the doses in spite of the improvement would say that, even though they felt much better or even though they became completely alright with the first few doses, yet to be on the safe side they finished off all the remaining powders. To my surprise, I did not find in these cases any dire consequences as I had been warned to expect. The acute disease was not aggravated nor did the symptoms return if they had ceased and the patient continued to remain well in spite of the doses having been thus repeated unnecessarily and against my orders. In fact, these patients appeared to have recovered quicker! In not a single case do I remember to have noted that the acute condition relapsed because the doses were repeated when not needed. On the other hand, the other group of patients, in whom the medicine was repeated only if and when absolutely necessary, i.e. only if and when they felt worse, seemed to take a longer time to come round. These were the patients who followed my instructions strictly and discontinued the doses, perhaps too soon. Thus I was gradually led to the conclusion that acute disease at least require more repetition of doses and that, at least in acute conditions, frequent repetition or repetition of doses, even when "not required", does not do any harm. Now, we come to the repetition of doses in chronic diseases.

Repetition in chronic cases: In chronic diseases, there are two standard procedures. In one, repeated doses of a low potency of the remedy are given till the patient is cured. In the other, a single dose of high potency is administered and then a wait follows till its action is over, *Sac-l* being given in the meanwhile.

Repetition of low potencies: The frequent repetition of low potencies in chronic conditions seems to be generally acceptable. For instance, for hard tumours, *Calc-f 6x* given two or three times a day for several weeks or months is quite a common prescription though it must be mentioned that people like R.T. Cooper were curing even chronic cases like peptic ulcers or even cancer with single doses of the medicine.

The real difference of opinion and disagreement seem to rise only about the frequent repetition of high potencies in chronic cases.

Repetition of high potencies: Going back to the teaching of Hahnemann, one is at first rather confused. Hahnemann in his teaching, upto and including the fourth edition of the *Organon*, has strictly warned against hasty repetition. We are advised not to repeat the dose until the effect of the previous dose is exhausted. In the 5th edition, he emphasizes this but there is a hint of a change. He mentions that "... this minutest yet powerful dose of the best selected medicine be repeated at suitable intervals." Later, in the preface to the third part of the 2nd edition of the *"Chronic Diseases"*, he says: "... in chronic disease I have found it best to allow a dose (to wit, a spoonful) of such a solution of the appropriate medicine to be taken no seldomer than every two days, but more generally every day."

This teaching is finally incorporated in the 6th edition and he writes, "The same carefully selected medicine may now be given daily for months..."

No doubt, Hahnemann's clear advice in the 5th edition, that a remedy should be repeated only when the effect of the previous dose has been completely exhausted, was implicity obeyed and the wisdom of this teaching repeatedly confirmed by his great followers like Allen, Boger, Clarke, Dunham, Farrington, Kent, Lippe, and many others. But we must remember that these masters did not have access to the later teachings of Hahnemann. They knew that Hahnemann was making some radical changes in his methods but since the 6th edition of the *Organon* was not published till as late as 1921 - thanks to the intransigence of Madame Melanie Hahnemann - though it was ready as early as in 1842, these masters had no idea about the new methods. They naturally faithfully followed and endorsed the original teachings of Hahnemann proposed and practised by him earlier, so that the final teachings of Hahnemann went unknown and therefore untested, unpractised and unendorsed.

During the 88 years that had lapsed between the publication of the 5th and 6th editions of the *Organon*, the teachings of Hahnemann as found in the 5th edition held the field, and it was natural that his great followers emphasized his teachings as contained in that edition. So when the latest edition came out in 1921, these new teachings apparently went against the weighty opinions of Kent and others and it was natural that no one seriously attempted to try them out.

Here, it would be worthwhile to go over the opinions, impressions and experiences of various well-known homoeopaths, as recorded in our literature.

Grisselich, after describing how Hahnemann had changed his idea about repetition in 1832 and had allowed earlier repetition, mentions that among his followers Aegidi was in favour of more frequent repetition. Also Tricks, Wolf, Gross, Kretshmar, Rau, Koempfer and Attomyr were all of similar opinion. Hering liked to repeat on the 2nd, 4th, 7th, 11th or 16th day, and until reaction or new symptoms appeared.

Ad. von Lippe (as quoted by Yingling) advises, where no response has been obtained, to repeat a lower potency in water every two hours till a good response is obtained, even if several days are required, and then to wait on its action. The single dose is an ideal dose but it is only applicable with the true similimum which is very difficult to get owing to the masked symptoms through promiscuous drugging. The farther removed the remedy is from the similimum, the greater must be the repetition to get necessary action upon which to wait for a cure or a change.

Baker says that one powder dry on the tongue may be all that is necessary, but again it is better to give three powders an hour apart or to dissolve a powder in six or ten teaspoonfuls of water and give two teaspoonfuls every half hour. Sometimes he gives one powder a day for three days or a powder night and morning for three days. But he never used this last method with potencies above the 200th.

Bellokossy considers that the wrong remedy has always some bad effect though only temporary. The high potencies produce much worse effects than the low. He also thinks that repetition of the dose will generally make the bad effects manifest. He further notes that he began to prescribe MM and potencies much higher than MM repeated once or twice a day for weeks and months. The results surpassed all expectations and produced infinitely better results. He also mentions that in acute cases you have to repeat but it is not necessary to plus. The same potency will be just as good.

Beronville says, "As a rule we must stop repeating as soon as we have effect from the medicine applied", and then suggests a new method which he says he has found very useful in his long experience. Repeat the dose, in however high dilution it may be, at short intervals until its action becomes apparent or give a high dilution and interpolate it with a lower one and stop the medicine as soon as its action is manifested and as long as it continues to act. If the amelioration is not complete, repeat in the same way.

Berridge feels that some cases, chronic or acute, may be cured by a single dose; others will require a repetition. The cases which need repetition are: (1) those to which no absolutely perfect similimum can be found and (2) those in which external disturbing factors continue to operate.

Blackley reports two cases of hydrocephalus treated with *Hellebore 1x* given persistently for months.

Boger opines that the repetition of doses is one of the most difficult subjects that the beginner can possibly handle. In case of a disease like malaria, a disease which inherently has the habit of recurring, he has never cured it with a single dose, especially if it were chronic. In such cases he gives a dose night and morning until he sees some effect, then stops and waits to see how long that effect is going to last. He goes on say, "In the case of a disease where it does not give an immediate effect, I am in favour of giving the highest potency in a single dose and then waiting a long time, as in the case of a miasm although I would not give the so-called anti-psorics for that purpose." Then he mentions that in slow, progressive diseases like arthritis deformans, it would be a mistake to prescribe a remedy and expect quick action because these diseases have a tendency to repeat and reassert their symptoms. In prescribing and administering the medicine, we have got to take into consideration the pace - the natural pace of the disease. Then he further mentions that he has sometimes waited three months for a reaction. But he notes that sometimes repetition is necessary particularly of the newer remedies, e.g. *Pyrogenum*. He also says that an aggravation from a high potency can be avoided by giving the remedy in three doses two hours apart.

Bradshaw thinks the failures to cure by high dilution are due to frequent repetition.

Buchmann says that he has often noticed aggravation from too frequent repetition and that he has frequently injured his patients by such undue haste. He says also that many remedies, e.g. *Bryonia, Belladonna*, etc., when properly selected, frequently show an improvement after the first dose. On repeating the dose, after some hours, an aggravation ensues at once, which increases more and more with every successive dose. So he never gives these remedies more often than twice a day even in acute cases.

Pulford thinks one may have to repeat the dose until it starts acting.

Campbell reports a case of *Bar. carb.* in which the 200th potency was given but did not relieve in a noticeably short time. Nevertheless, he persisted in giving it at four-hour-intervals for a number of weeks and got results. He feels that in an aged person the vitality may need many doses to gather sufficient momentum to carry the patient to a complete cure.

G.H. Clarke considers that Hahnemann's dictum must be observed, viz. that the dose should not be repeated while the amelioration lasts.

Coleman says that the secret of Burnett's successes lay in the infrequent repetition of the dose. This gave the body a chance to react. Infrequent repetition is the successful method of treatment by isopathy or vaccine therapy, today.

Cooper strongly advises us to rely on a single and solitary dose, even if it is one drop of the O. He quotes the case of deafness of four years cured by a single dose of *Mez.* given by Dunham. He calls repetition "a barbarous habit". He also describes a case of skin disease in which he prescribed *Calc. carb. 3x* t.d.s. The patient reported after six months that he was completely cured, not while taking the medicines, but three weeks after stopping it. So, Cooper decided to rely hence forth more than ever upon the single dose, and to allow a sufficient time to pass before repeating the dose. Since then, he says, his success proved to be much greater.

Dhawale says, "In chronic cases, I generally use the single dose. In resistant cases, repeated doses of the same potency or in the ascending potency scale are employed to the point of reaction. In acute diseases, I repeat often till a definite response is obtained and then I cut down progressively on the frequency as improvement sets in."

Dienst reports a case where he gave *Carbol. acid 30*, 4 hourly at least for 2 weeks.

Dixon is against repeating the dose too early.

Edward Philips considers that the rightly selected remedy will cure more effectively when given at distant intervals.

Ewart writes, "High potencies are in some homoeopathic circles spoken of almost with bated breath. I do not know whether this is due to the famous warning by Dr. Kent: "It is well to realise that you are dealing with razors when dealing with the high potencies. I would rather be in a room with a dozen negros slashing with razors than in the hands of an ignorant prescriber of high potencies. They are the means of tremendous harm as well as of tremendous good." (Kent's Lectures, p. 453). This warning is calculated to make the beginner steer clear of high potencies for the rest of his life. It is however hardly couched in the cool language of science and may have been due to an unfortunate experience of the doctor giving a homoeopathic remedy to a moribund patient. When the lamp of life is burning low, the exhibition of a homoeopathic remedy, high or low, is probably like a gust of wind. There is a last flicker, then extinction. At all events, in most quarters, high potencies are usually given at rare intervals. You can however find instances in homoeopathic books of cases where the CM potency has been repeated daily. I have done so myself on suitable patients, and nothing but good has resulted. Daily repetition in a sensitive patient should be avoided as it produces on excited restless state.

"Although high potencies are used sparingly, most homoeopaths are more lavish with lower potencies, even in chronic diseases. Common sense would seem to suggest that if the frequent repetition of high potencies is dangerous, then the frequent use of lower potencies is more dangerous since the lower potencies contain many million times the quantity compared with the higher potencies. As lower potencies can apparently be repeated t.d.s. with impunity, why cannot high potencies? I have made such experiments on myself with the CM potency over the past few years with so far no untoward results, in fact with benefit. For example, two hard tumours on the right side of my nasal septum, which practically blocked the right nostril, have gradually reduced in size. They had been in existence some 20 years before the homoeopathic treatment.

"The rule I have tentatively adopted in giving high potencies, which I find more curative than low, is to dissolve the pilules in about 8 oz of water, and give a tablespoonful as a dose, instructing the patient to wait 10 days or so for reaction; if no reaction to repeat daily until reaction (aggravation or improvement) appears when the doses should be stopped, the dose not to be repeated until improvement comes to an end."

Fraser Kerr reports a case where he gave *Bry. 1 M* in plussed doses daily for forty-nine consecutive days.

Gagliardi mentions having prescribed *Nat-m 30* seven doses, one dose every 3rd day for a patient.

George Royal quotes several cases - one of a child with a tumour on the head half the size of an egg for which he gave *Calc-c 30* daily once for 2 weeks and than occasionally. For another similar case, he gave *Lapis alba 12*, twice a day for 3 weeks and then intermittently.

Gordon believes that Dishington's discovery of plus dosage, "has proved its value beyond all question or cavil". He has long used the single dose and for the last two years has been experimenting with double dosage. "This consists in giving, instead of the familiar single dose, two doses of different potencies, 24 hours or 48 hours apart, e.g. *Phos. 200* (1) followed in 24 hours time by *Phos. 1M* (1). Thereafter, treatment proceeds exactly as for single doses except that instead of *Sac-l* (1), one gives two doses *Sac-l* 24 hours apart." Gordon holds that this method, in his experience, applies only to chronic diseases; that it is particularly useful in cases in which the single dose has failed to give results both deeper and quicker; that the average duration of action is usually, but not always shorter, ranging from about six to eight weeks that it is more profitable to repeat the double dosage in the same potencies at the second prescription and go higher for the third and fourth and higher again for the fifth and sixth; that the lower potencies are more effective when the patients's vitality is low; that the double dose causes harm instead of good in cases of deficient vitality. He believes, with Blunt, that plus dosage is of little value for potencies above 30, also, that when double fails, esp. among neurasthenics, triple dosage may be effectively given as follows: *Nit-ac 1M*, one dose, then 48 hrs later *Nit-ac 10M*, one dose and again 48 hrs later *Nit-ac 45 M*, one dose.

Grimmer while discussing Hahnemann's "New and Improved Method of Repetition" says, "Kent did say you could give in acute cases, the medicine in repeated doses, and he did it especially in febrile cases."

Harish Chand quotes Kamfor who suggested the repetition of remedies in increasing amount.

Hayes thinks that there is one serious objection to giving repeated doses, and that is late aggravation esp. in chronic cases. He had seen quite severe aggravation occur several weeks - as many as twelve weeks - after good improvement.

Horace Reed endorses the method of infrequent repetition in chronic cases.

Houghton reports his method of repetition. He says that he has given nearly all the long-acting remedies in several hundred cases, a single remedy at a time night and morning for four days at a time followed by another similar remedy for 4 days or a week and so on for 3 to 6 months. Alternatively, he used to select four or five of the most strictly appropriate remedies for a given case, each one covering as many symptoms as possible, and administer one dose of each remedy during a day (that is four or five doses in all) for seven successive days then to give single remedies, night and morning for four days and after a week, to repeat the series of five medicines, daily for another week, and so on for a month or two*. He further says, "For my own part, being largely engaged in the treatment of chronic diseases, many of my patients being at a distance and never personally seen, I have indulged in the use of very low dilutions, tinctures, first triturations, and even crude drugs, and have repeated these remedies oftener than the strict homoeopathic rules permit, without being disturbed by aggravations and with a degree of success, which leads me to think that some writers are far too timid and fastidious in regard to doses and repetitions."

Hubbard describes how she repeated the dose in a case expecting the patient to be worse but he got better, "I was giving it in one dose. It seemed to me he was not getting well on the one dose. I am afraid I was just plain experimenting with that 30. I went to see him carefully. After he had had the four doses, if he had been worse, I would have stopped it instantly. He appeared to get better. I told his wife to stop it instantly if he appeared to get worse, at any moment, but he fooled us and got gradually better, so I am afraid I have no reason for it except God given despair." But she teaches generally a single dose. She quotes Borland's claim that frequently he pulls through the pneumonias with a single dose. She further says, "I knew Borland when I studied over there thirty years ago, and admired him immensely. I have never seen any results from this so-called plussing, just a few shakes and pounds on your hand. I never have liked that."

John Weir thinks the rate of repetition is dependent entirely on the response of the patient. He quotes a case of *Sulph.* in which the patient was given a single dose to which he did not respond for 3 weeks but responded very well to it in the 4th week.

Johnson considers the best thing to do is to wait.

Julian says that if experience shows that regular repetition is more beneficial we need not blindly follow Hahnemann.

Writing on the subject of repetition, Kanjilal emphasizes giving a single dose and waiting until the action of the single dose is definitely finished. He gives examples of cases spoiled by undue repetition. He quotes a case in which *Ars. alb.* 6x gave relief to the patient for six months and another case where a dose of *Sulph.* 10M repeated to hasten the action of *Sulph.* 200 given earlier produced a fatal effect. He also describes another case in which a patient given *Lyc.* 200 did not find any effect for three weeks but then started improving. But, by mistake, he took a dose of *Sulph.* 200 and this made him worse and it took more than six months to repair the damage. He says, "From the very beginning to the end we never prescribe more than one or two doses of the indicated medicine and observe reaction for weeks or sometimes months, never thinking of repetition or a second prescription so long as there is the slightest trace of the continued action of the previous dose. It is an irrefutable fact of experience of all, that as soon as there is any evidence of reaction of the previous dose or doses, further medication must be stopped until the reaction is completely over." Commenting on Maganlal Desai's, "adventurous" repetition of high potencies, he further says that he has an open mind on the question and feels that this frequent repetition method cannot be accepted until there is more strong objective evidence in its favour.

Kostenlitz is of the same opinion as Julian.

Le Hunte Cooper says that in his experience remedies in the 30th potency can be repeated every 3rd day while 100C and 200C will act satisfactorily at intervals of a week though much longer than this may, in special cases, be required for either. He personally had not found any adverse effects from such frequent repetition.

Mahony writes that *Calc-c* can be repeated frequently in children but not in the adults or the aged...

McLaren reports a case of rheumatic fever for which he gave *Lachesis MM* for five nights successively with very rapid improvement. He also records that Terril used to give two or three doses of the 200th potency everyday for a week or two with some wonderful results.

Mohan Singh strongly advises against indiscriminate repetition and quotes cases which were harmed by such rapid repetition.

Phatak, the veteran homoeopath, says that in his experience, more frequent repetition of doses seems to be needed nowadays than used to be needed some 20 or 30 years back. Possibly patients are exposed to more stresses and strains and other morbid influences; possibly they transgress the laws of nature more than before; perhaps foods are devitalised or contaminated, perhaps the atmosphere is disturbed by industrial or radioactive material. But whatever the reasons, the effect of the medicine seems to be less long-lasting. So there does seem to be a case for more frequent repetition.

Pulford notes that he has seen excellent result with the single dose and thinks that the dose should be repeated only if its action is interfered with by some other cause. He advises even in acute cases such as pneumonia, a single dose of the 200th and cautions never to repeat until one is absolutely sure that the previous dose has ceased to act. But he also thinks that one may have to repeat the dose until it sticks, then any further dose will be superfluous.

Puddephatt says that low potencies like the 3rd and 12th can be repeated two or three times a day. The higher you go, the less often must the remedy be given.

Quinton records that, in cases of high B.P., he might give remedies like *Sulph., Bar-c, etc. 30, daily.* He further states that the average duration of action of 30th potency is a week or fortnight and that the 200 could be repeated certainly after 20 days. He feels it worthwhile to experiment and see if the patient would do better with the more frequent repetition of high potency. He also feels there is a tendency to leave the repetition of the doses too long whether they were light, medium or low potency. Referring to Hahnemann's teaching not to repeat the dose often, Quinton says he would disagree with him and no doubt many other homoeopaths would join him in disagreeing. He writes, "If a statement is incorrect and can be shown to be incorrect by experiments, then it really does not matter how great the man was who made the statement."

Rabe in his editorial notes describes a case of a woman who was suffering for 6 weeks from tearing pain in back. He gave her *Rhus-t 30* four times each day, for six days, at the end of which she was decidedly better. So he then gave her *Rhus-t 200*, thrice a day for another six days and then found that she improved further.

Reed thinks it is a fatal error to repeat the dose too soon either in acute or chronic cases.

Ross writes that at the opposite extreme we have recent syphilis which, as Hahnemann pointed out, requires repetition of the homoeopathic remedy several times a day in physiological dosage, gradually diminishing the crude amounts of drug with potentizing as cure proceeds. In fact, he thinks that all illness due to continued active infection, with fever and high E.S. R., require frequent repetition of the remedy in water with minor changes of potency as advised in the 6th edition of the *Organon* until improvement is very obvious. He further quotes a case of sciatica in the hospital in which he had to repeat Tuberculinum 4 or 5 times within a month.

Senseman says that when you want to prevent something, say a patient is under the continuous possibility of exposure to a contagion - just one or two doses will not suffice. They must be given for a lengthy period.

Shirtliff records that Holcombe prescribed for a case of suspected tuberculosis *Calc-c 200*, daily one dose for 3 months.

Stewart mentions that Burnett used to repeat *Bacillinum* once a week.

Sutherland says that weeks and frequently months will lapse before it becomes necessary to give a second dose of the chosen remedy. It is remarkable too, how well these cases get along in the meanwhile.

Tomlinson writes that Lippe used to give one dose of high potency and would even wait for six months before giving the second dose. He reports that in a very serious case seen in consultation with Moore and H.N. Guernsey, he had selected the indicated remedy the giving of which was followed by prompt improvement. Then turning to his conferrers he said, "Gentlemen, whatever you do, do not give the patient another dose; if you do, she will die." Some time after Lippe had gone, however, the temptation became too great to resist and they did repeat the dose. The woman died promptly as prophesied.

Among the high potency prescribers also, Tyler was in the habit of giving 3 doses every 2 hours and then following it with Sac-l. She had the impression that such repetition at short intervals cuts down the aggravation if any. S.R. Phatak, C.C. Desai and others like them administer the dose 2 or 3 times a day till the effect becomes apparent and then they withhold their hands as long as this improvement continues. This dose can be called the single cumulative dose as against the single dose. The object is to get a single cumulative effect.

Others also have experienced and noted the need for frequent repetition. Wilson writes, "Repetition appears to me to be more often necessary than it used to be. Here, I am generalising with other than skin troubles in mind." He quotes Borland as saying that in modern life, we would need to repeat much more often.

Wilson describes a case of bronchitis where he had to repeat *Tuberculinum* every fortnight.

Woodbury records that in dropsies of general origin *Arsen.*, *Samb.*, or whatever remedy is indicated will, if used in the 30th to the 200th potency and repeated frequently several days and renewed when necessary, sweep out the fluid with great relief. He thinks that there might be cases in which a single dose might not suffice and that several repetitions might be needed.

Yingling says that it is thought dangerous to repeat *Lachesis* especially in high potencies, yet Berridge of London, reports a case cured by the repetition of *Lachesis MM*, night and morning for one whole week. He then quotes what Kent had written to him some years earlier, that in low fevers it was usually necessary to repeat the dose even every two or three hours for days before getting the required impression of the drug essential for a speedy and complete cure. He writes, "These illustrations are made to prove that the crude drug will cure when selected according to the law of cure. But it will be noticed that the drug is necessarily repeated most frequently, even every fifteen to thirty minutes for day, then one or two hours for other days bordering on weeks even when the patient is better and the drug's action has been quite marked. While these cases were cured with the crude drug, they could have been cured more promptly and with less suffering and expense by the use of a potency from the 200th upward."

Apart from the fact that no new methods have been considered or tried out, no experiment of any sort worth mentioning has been attempted. It must be admitted further with surprise that even the teaching of Hahnemann as found in the 6th edition of the *Organon* which differs materially from his original teachings as contained in the previous editions of the book have not been put into practice. Homoeopaths in general have shown a great reluctance to try out these methods. As an excuse for this hesistancy it has even been suggested by some that these latest teachings are the outcome of a senile brain of the Master and therefore valueless. These statements are not only unsubstantiated and unfair, but also unfortunate because Hahnemann has always appealed that all his ideas should be put to the test of practice. It would therefore be a pity if we, his followers, should condemn his teachings without testing, a fault which we find with our allopathic colleagues with reference to Homoeopathy. Hahnemann had evolved and practised this method of frequent repetition after he shifted to Paris, and it gains still more respect because it was in Paris that he became most successful and had the largest clientele. In fact his phenomenal success in Paris might have been due to the developments and modifications of his original methods. He himself writes very approvingly about these new methods.

Sankaran reports that, considering firstly that nothing should be condemned without test; secondly that Hahnemann had clearly emphasized that his new method was born of further experience and that it had proved to be superior; and thirdly that Kent and others had no inkling at all that such a new method had been propounded by Hahnemann and therefore, had no opportunity to try them out and compare the results, he decided to put this new method to the test. Further, even though the 6th edition had not been published then at least one homoeopath in the shape of George Royal had envisaged such a practice.

He wrote: "I should like to emphasize one point which I think is hardly appreciated by the younger men. When I left college, I went out with the impression that the application of the remedy should be more frequent in acute than in chronic diseases; that the acute disease was like an enemy that must be overcome by many charges before he would take himself away. The chronic disease on the other hand was supposed to be like an enemy entrenched but asleep, where the attack need not be repeated to overcome him. My actual experience is to the contrary and I believe that the remedy needs more frequent repetition in the chronic disease."

In order to test the results of the frequent repetition of high potencies in chronic diseases, to know whether they benefit or do harm, Sankaran conducted a number of experiments in the Government Homoeopathic Hospital, Bombay. Whereas the original practice had been to stop the medicine as soon as any effect became noticeable whether as a result of the single dose or the collective dose - the single effect being the aim - he started very gradually and cautiously repeating the medicine even when some improvement was evident as a result of the previous dose. Having satisfied himself that such frequent repetition did not bring about any untoward results, he slowly reached the stage of repeating the doses daily. A number of cases were put under the new schedule of dosage, the potencies varying with each case ranging from the 6th to the CM. He was carefully watching out for any unpleasant reactions but he noted only three cases which showed such reactions and which had hitherto responded very well to the unit dose.

To selected cases he administered the indicated medicine in high potencies repeatedly and did not find any harmful effects. For instance, he reports that in a case of convulsions in which the remedy indicated was *Cup. met.*, the patient was given one dose of *Cup. 200*. There was an immediate improvement which lasted 3 months. Then he had relapses at intervals and every time he was given *Cup.* at intervals in single doses as follows: 1M after 10 days; 10M after 63 days and 8 days; 50M after 55 days and 67 days; CM after 73 days and 35 days. He showed improvement with every repetition. Then, from 01.12.58 onwards as an experiment he was given *Cup. met. 30*, once daily for a week, then from 08.12.58, 200, once daily, from 06.01.59, 1M, daily once and from 27.07.59, CM, daily once upto 05.08.59. The effect of such repetition was in no way deleterious and the patient became practically normal.

He then gives some more illustrative cases.

Cases

1. A patient Mr. P.N., aged 30 years, was admitted to the hospital on June 11, 1957, with a history of oedema of the lower limbs, puffiness of the face and oliguria of five years duration, with intermittent remissions and exacerbation. His case was taken thoroughly and all investigations done and a diagnosis of hypoproteinemia was arrived at. The symptoms indicated the probable similimum as *China ars.*

Therefore, the patient was put on *Chi-a 200*, t.d.s. whereupon his urine output which originally averaged 6 to 8 oz per day gradually and steadily rose to 78 oz per day within a fortnight. The puffiness and oedema considerably lessened. However, despite the steady rise in the urinary output and the proportionate improvement in the general condition, the medicine was continuously repeated and despite the repetition the improvement continued. Whenever the response to the drug lessened the potency was merely changed, being usually raised or sometimes lowered, whereupon the response increased. The patient was kept under observation for six months and in all during this period he received doses of *China ars.* as mentioned below.

6th potency, 87 doses; 12th potency, 14 doses; 30th potency, 65 doses; 200th potency, 14 doses; 1000th potency, 25 doses.

On December 13, 1957, he was discharged as completely relieved.

2. Mrs. K.A., aged 30, was admitted on September 28, 1957, for paraplegia of one year's duration. She had incontinence of urine and stool and flaccid paralysis of the lower limbs. She complained of heaviness of the body, stitching pains in all the joints, heaviness alternating with tingling and burning of the lower limbs, burning of the soles, etc. She was brought into the hospital on a stretcher. Her case worked out to *Causticum*, and she was put on this remedy. There was an immediate and remarkable improvement even with the first few doses but the administration of the remedy was continued nevertheless. In all she stayed in the hospital for three months after which time she walked out, completely

relieved. During this period she received *Causticum* as described below:

1M potency, 27 doses; 10M potency, 28 doses; CM potency, 15 doses.

No ill effect of any sort was noticed at any time.

Among the many subacute and chronic cases treated in this manner were cases of chronic bronchitis, bronchial asthma, eczema, paralysis, pulmonary tuberculosis, nephritis, papillomata, psoriasis, carbuncle, etc. Only in the three cases, as mentioned earlier some aggravation was noticed that could be attributed to the repetition. Of course, only about a hundred cases had been put on this schedule of dose during a period of one year and so both the number of cases and the period of observation are insufficient to come to any conclusion. But this much can be said that the original rule put forward by many homoeopaths that repetition of the medicine done while the effect of the previous dose is still evident will invariably do harm and that such repetition would retard the progress is perhaps not justified in all cases as judged by the limited experience quoted above. If the rule holds good at all, then it must be recorded that many exceptions were met with! Incidentally, Hahnemann has clearly mentioned that only potencies of his new LM scale should be repeated. So, Sankaran as also Ramanlal Patel have independently tried out repetition of these potencies and found beneficial effects from such dosage. According to the original methods of repetition of dosage taught by Hahnemann in the 5th and previous editions of the *Organon*, we are to give infrequent doses of the appropriate medicine in the appropriate potency. Each such dose is expected to produce a mild imperceptible aggravation followed by an amelioration. The dose was to be repeated only when the amelioration ceases. As per the new teaching in the 6th edition of the *Organon*, we are allowed to give even daily doses of the medicine in chronic disease, doses of the LM potencies, every subsequent dose being a slightly higher potency than the previous dose. These doses are expected to produce no aggravation, but only a continuous amelioration till cure is established. But when a cure is established the further repetition of the doses produce a recurrence of symptoms or aggravation. Then medication is stopped and the patient becomes normal. The process of cure by these two methods can be represented graphically as follows:

New Method of Repetition - *Organon* 6th edition

Further careful experimentation by other independent observers will, no doubt, confirm or contradict these conclusions and will no doubt, reveal the fact whether repetition of the medicine while the patient is improving is actually harmful, harmless or beneficial.

In recent times in our country, practitioners like Maganbhai Desai, Sarabhai Kapadia, Kripal Singh Baxi and several others have reported various cases in which the indicated remedy has been frequently repeated in high potencies with beneficial results. Particularly a series of cases of pulmonary tuberculosis, some even with cavities in the lungs, reported by Maganbhai Desai is noteworthy.

Now let us look at another aspect of the picture. First, it must be recorded that such rapid repetition of high potencies is not generally practised by the homoeopathic profession at large. On the other hand, they are taught to repeat only when the dose is absolutely needed again, if at all. So, notwithstanding the reported experiences, illustrations and arguments, such frequent administration of high potencies, e.g. the repeated administration of CM potencies, four times a day for four months as was done in a chronic case*, is at first bound to evoke a feeling of misgiving, fear or even alarm in the minds of orthodox homoeopathic practitioners. Homoeopathic practitioners, by and large, follow the techniques and precepts of Kent and most of them usually adhere, in chronic cases at least, to the method of giving a single dose of high potency of the homoeopathic remedy and repeating it at long intervals as and when necessary. Alternatively they administer low potencies more frequently. Almost all the galaxy of past masters from Hahnemann downwards to Sir John Weir and Pierre Schmidt (including Allen, Boenninghausen, Boger, Dunham, Farrington, Kent, Lippe, etc.) have advised against frequent and unnecessary repetition of high potencies. Some of them think it can actually obstruct the cure.

There is also the cardinal principle of Homoeopathy which expounds the use of minimum doses. The homoeopath believes that the sick organism requires only the minimal stimulus to overcome the illness and to return to its original normal state. Roberts says that the dose should be diluted in time as well as in space, meaning thereby that the dose should not be given frequently. He says further that the successful homoeopath knows how and when to wait. He also mentions that to do this, i.e. to hold one's hand, is the hardest thing for a physician to do and the really successful homoeopath will be the one who can do so. He, like the obstetrician, must know the secret of "watchful expectancy and masterly inactivity". Besides, if a minimum dose can cure why should we give the maximum number of doses? Maximum doses and frequent repetition are more commonly associated with the allopathic method of treatment. This is the view of most homoeopaths. Hahnemann himself has praised the value of sugar of milk, calling it "a gift" meaning thereby that the judicious use of this placebo instead of the medicine can be most beneficial.

In spite of this concept which we have inherited, imbibed and confirmed, and which to us forms one of the pillars of Homoeopathy, we have to consider the experiences and claims of Desai and others, and see if their method of prescribing is superior to or an advancement on the single dose technique in anyway, for example, whether it hastens the cure of the patient. Unfortunately sufficient objective statistical data are not available by which we can form valid conclusions. No doubt the cases reported by these homoeopaths have been treated successfully with such rapid repetition of high potencies. But there is no comparative presentation and study of cases treated with infrequent repetition and similar ones treated by frequent repetition of high potencies to prove that the latter method is indeed infinitely superior and quicker in its action.

Now again, the question will arise whether such frequent repetition of high potencies is harmful or not. There is the possibility that in sensitive patients, it may actually give rise to more symptoms of the same remedy which the innocent or ignorant prescriber may consider as clear indications for the further doses of the same drug. Sensitive patients may be aggravated, sometimes even badly, by the repeated administration of high potencies. We have known of cases in which the patients were violently upset by the repeated dose of even moderate and low potencies. Again, we have to consider the possibility, however remote, that some of the patients who took such treatment might have felt worse and therefore discontinued the treatment without the physician being aware of these results. This possibility must be considered since all the patients were not treated in an indoor hospital.

Therefore, it would seem rash to start prescribing CM potency three or four times a day in chronic cases indiscriminately for every case! At best, such a practice can be followed, if at all, only by an experienced prescriber and cautious physician who is completely aware of what he is doing and who can carefully interpret and control the effects and if necessary neutralise the ill-effects of such repetition. In the hands of the large majority of less experienced homoeopathic practitioners, who may not be able to assess things so carefully, this method can prove to be dangerous and the results absolutely disastrous for the patient and the physician.

It may not be, therefore, advisable for the large majority of less experienced homoeopathic practitioners to adopt this method straightway. It would be preferable to conduct carefully controlled trials and note the advantages or disadvantages of this method before adopting it universally (P Sankaran 1996).

Chapter Nine | Best Practice, Potency and Administration

In this chapter you will:
1. Understand the context of choice of potency
2. Read the best practice directives of different authors
3. Critically think about their value

Chapter 9

Best Practice, Potency and Administration

9.1 The Luck of the Draw

A lot depends upon who your primary teacher is or was. They are always right, right? This is what I was taught when it came to posology. For years, this is also what I taught students. The choice of potency depends on the proximity to the simillimum. Roberts argued the greater number of characteristic symptoms of the disease that were to be found to correspond to the homeopathic remedy, the less the quantity and higher the potency can be used (Roberts 1936). Then there is the intensity of the disease expression. Another consideration is the predominance of mental or physical disease expression. This is the idea often articulated that physical symptoms need a low potency. Further, when mental symptoms are clear it is better to start with 200 or higher. Then there is the nature of the condition. This is the idea that advanced physical pathological conditions do not lend themselves to high potencies. In suppressed conditions, skin complaints etc. it is better not to start with high potencies. Aggravation is always a possibility. In Addition to all that, we must take into account the sensitivity of the individual. Elderly people and those that are convalescing or frail, who are debilitated are better to start on low potencies. When it comes to hypersensitive individuals for whom any contact with colour, sounds, movies, music, energy, people, parties, television elicit an intense reaction, it is better to start with a conservative medium potency and a test dose. Children and infants vitality is usually stronger and therefore a higher potency is more easily integrated.

It all sounds so clear and easy.

9.2 Burnett on Potency

There were a couple of reasons it dawned on me over the years that not all that was written above made perfect sense to me. The idea of selecting a high potency based on my own levels of confidence and 'being a mental case' was simply not my experience in the clinic, nor from having conducted a number of provings. I was talking to some students about it one day. Surprisingly one of them wrote me an email the next day

> Dear Mr Gray,
>
> Here are two statements I found. My previous boss lent me some books which I read randomly in the dispensary last time. Anyway I suppose most people will belittle the high potency as in Dr. Burnett's term.
>
> The greater to similitude the higher the dilution and the less frequent the administration; the smaller the degree of similitude and lower the dose and the more frequent the repetition of the dose. Burnett, Fifty Reasons for being a Homoeopath.

I would summarize the whole thing thus: Where the organ-ailing is primary to the organ, use organ remedies in little material doses frequently repeated; where the organ-ailing is of piece pathologically with that of the organism, use the homeopathic simillimum in high potency infrequently repeated. (Burnett 1888).

9.3 Kent's Flexibility and the Endless Field

It is worthwhile reading what Kent wrote on the issue of the selection of potency. He was clearly not well when he made this address but it highlights flexibility and is free from the dogmatism of which he is often accused.

Kent: Observations regarding the selection of the potency

I must apologise to the association for not having written a paper, but I have been too tired and too ill to prepare one; I made the mistake of putting its preparation off too long, until when College closed I had a little break-down and since I have not been able to write a paper, I will, however, make a verbal report.

The question of what is the best potency for a given case and the question of what is the potency that is best for habitual use is a broad subject. When I was a boy, I played with chicken's feet when they were being prepared for the family dinner and it was my first study in anatomy. I found that by pulling certain tendons or strings as I called them, that the corresponding toes would double up. Every one of the toes could be made to contract by pulling certain strings but it was a very clumsy motion compared with the natural orderly movements of the toes when they were on the chicken. This leads me to jump a long way, to say that I have been in the office of many homoeopathic physicians who have in their armamentarium nothing but tinctures, and I think that that is clumsier than pulling the strings to make the chicken's toes move.

I have been in other physician's offices where nothing could be found but CMs. In my opinion, that too was a somewhat arbitrary selection; it showed a partiality for a certain potency that was too arbitrary and not sufficiently based upon judgment. There is a wonderful latitude between the tinctures and the CMs and in my judgment the selection of the best potency is a matter of experience and observation and not as yet a matter of law.

There is an almost endless field here for speculation and observation, ranging from the tinctures to the highest potencies, with the possibility of bringing out some useful rules for the guidance of others. The various potencies are all more or less related to individuals and it is the individual that we should study. We might well begin with Hahnemann's statement that the 30 is low enough or strong enough to begin with. For many years I have found it strong enough to begin with. Individualization, in regard to potencies as in other branches of homoeopathic work, furnishes us with an additional element of accuracy and success, enabling us to reach certain cases that we otherwise could not reach. Some patients are very sensitive to the highest potencies and are cured mildly and permanently by the use of the 200th or 1000th. There are other individuals who are torn to pieces by the use of the highest potencies.

The indiscriminate use of any one potency is very likely to bring reproach upon our art. They all, from the 30th to the millionth, have their place, but no single potency is equal to the demands made upon it by the diseases of different individuals. Then the nature of the disease makes a difference; patients who have heart disease, or who are suffering from phthisis are apt to have their sufferings increased and the end hastened by the highest potencies; they do better under the 30th or 200th. Sometimes very sensitive patients will do well on a high potency if they have been prepared for it by the use of a lower one. I have frequently seen patients recover from their symptoms for a while under the 1000th and then the remedy would cease to act. A repetition of it would be followed by no effect. The 10,000th would then produce a very beneficial effect and make the cure permanent. Give the necessary doses at long intervals until the repetition brings no effect; then if you are sure that it is the similimum give it in a higher potency until that ceases to act and finally the highest. In this way we can put a patient upon a series of potencies and keep up a prolonged curative action lasting for several years.

The prolonged action is sometimes necessary in very chronic deep-seated diseases. A few months would exhaust the action of a drug if only one potency was used. Any potency, no matter what it is, high or low, will cease to act after a time. That shows at once the usefulness of knowing about more than one single potency of a medicine. Hahnemann gave us an axiom in this respect; it was "when the remedy ceases to act, give a single dose of sulphur to awaken the susceptibility." This would not be so often necessary if the potency was properly varied. It was also more necessary with the earlier practitioners of homoeopathy because they had a limited number of medicines to handle compared to us. I have not used sulphur as an intercurrent for a long time because the indicated remedy will not so often cease to have a curative effect if the potency is properly varied.

I have been told by many homoeopathic physicians that they have used the 3rd, 6th or 12th, and obtained a fair result and then it ceased to act at all. Such prescribers have no range of potency and they fail to make a complete cure. Several times I have seen patients on repeated doses of the right remedy in a low potency make no improvement, simply because their susceptibility to that potency-not to that remedy by any means-had been exhausted. I have taken such patients and without changing the remedy but simply the potency got a curative result.

When a patient returns and upon examination you find the old symptoms still there although the patient says that he or she feels much better, that is not the time for repeating the dose. It is only a question of time when a cure will result. When a patient returns and says that he is losing ground, then it is the remedy that has ceased to act, not the potency. Now you need to hunt up another remedy and not a change of potency. Remember that these things are not as yet matters of law but simply the results of some observation. I have always been interested in experiments and observations upon this question, and there is a great deal of work for all of us to do in this field.

Of course it is only the men who hew close to the line that can furnish observations of value. I am always willing and glad to listen to such a man's experience with the greatest interest. One of the important uses of a society like this is to bring out the experience and observation of trained men such as make up the bulk of its members.

Potencies discussion

Question: What is the explanation of antidoting high potencies by using low ones? In tuberculosis, for instance, *Sulphur* is occasionally too deep-acting, and a less similar remedy may work up to a stronger totality so that better results may be possible.

Kent: The correspondence doctrine of series and degrees comes near to mastering the question of using potentization. The crude drug and the potentized remedy are opposite in action. In proving a remedy, of one of the elements that exists in the body (*Sulphur*, for instance, helps make up the body), the prover takes crude *Sulphur* until it produces a proving. He is unable then to appropriate it from the food to build up the body, being cloyed with it. The symptoms of the *Sulphur* patient indicate that she needs it, but she is not able to appropriate it from the food. Each resembles the other.

Give the patient with symptoms of *Sulphur* the potency; if you give it cruder than it is in the natural body, etc., it only makes her worse. The higher potency of *Sulphur* restores order and she appropriates it from the food, not being fed enough to poison her.

There are distinct degrees from the potency to the crude form; according to the excitability of the patient, she reacts to the 200, 500, 1000, and so on, these being only illustrative. If a given remedy will make an individual react and appropriate that which is needed and help to appropriate from the blood that which is taken, the reaction may be to 5M, and though not eaten it is in the blood.

Degrees are in sevens, as in octaves of music. If you strike too high she is not sensitive, it is not sufficient. Keep to the mild potency so long as it works. It is not well to jump too many degrees. From the crude to 10M there is a range of degrees in the ordinary person. You do not go from the first to the last, in music, it does not preserve the chord, you take the thirds and fifths. You can repeat the series, beginning with the lower potencies, and do good work.

The patient will recognize these series. Too high a potency gives an unnecessary aggravation, and then will not perform the best curative action. The best action is the slight aggravation, as in the first few hours in the acute disorders. The ideal is the one that gives no aggravation but amelioration. We do not seek to produce an aggravation, that is not the best, not the longest curative effect. No law is established for aggravations and ameliorations. Only by study of records in practical experience, can we see the best action in patients.

Question. Can you give too deep-acting potency to be curative; would a less similar give safer results?

Kent: The cruder approaches the opposite and antidotes; the low potencies approach in degrees to the higher potencies. In the *Sulph.* patient who needed *Sulphur* ten or twenty years ago, and today it would kill her; *Nux, Pulsatilla, Senega,* palliate but cure. I have seen *Sulph.* and *Phos.* act so strongly that I have regretted it. In lung cases, consider whether she has lung space enough to make recovery probable. If she can bear it, give it in a low potency, but do not give it if there is not lung space enough to warrant it.

Question. I have a mentally deficient child, whose mind becomes clearer every time I advance in the plane. She has had *Barium sulph.* It is an unusual case. Would you go to the bottom, and recommend the series, or higher to MM?

Kent: There you may be going into trouble and confusion. One patient may run up safely, but ninety-nine cases would not have any action in those high potencies. The object is to keep the patient under the influence of the remedy the longest time possible; to follow up with just enough difference to react, to reach the best-acting plane. From experience, I am led to use of a series from 1M to DM (5CM) including 10M, somewhere near 50M, and CM. Other potencies are given, to observe what action is forthcoming. You encourage the patient to become oversensitive by using the highest potencies, instead of going low to begin again. As a rule, two doses (sometimes three) in the same plane give the best results. It has become almost routine, as the records indicate that the third dose in the same potency gives no effect. It is a mistake to mix degrees and the different makes. If Allen, Ehrhart, or Kent's has been started, stick to the same series and the same scale.

Pure homoeopathy defended

"What can be more astonishing than that professed homoeopathic physicians should deny the efficacy of their own remedies?"

"What greater evidence can the public ask of ignorance of the system they profess to make use of to cure the sick?"

It has been known to many witnesses that I have not needed anything but homoeopathic remedies in incurables. I have been giving unusual attention to incurables, in private and hospital practice, where cancer and phthisis pains have been present, where morphine had, in other hands, entirely failed, and in all cases has the homoeopathic remedy, when properly selected, been all that was needed. Argument will fail to convince some physicians, for the reason that they cannot cure and they cannot be made to believe that anyone else can. They do not know how to palliate and they do not believe that anyone else knows. If they cannot cure, how then can they be expected to palliate or vice versa. You may freely say that for years I have offered to show that the severest sufferings from phthisis and cancer, can be subdued with potentized homoeopathic remedies. You may say that my students all do it, and say openly that we do not need anodynes. Let any man select cases of cancer or phthisis and bring them to the Woman's Homoeopathic Hospital, and bring his own judges, and we will teach him to palliate the most painful cases with the indicated remedy. We challenge the world to this very test. I might report cases and they would not be accepted, but there is the hospital that treats these cases and here is the place to see it done. We have now many cases of phthisis and some of cancer. A patient under my care who is being cured of a fibroid of the uterus, a tumor as large as her head, and she (the patient) is returning to health.

It is astonishing that physicians will not listen to men who know how to cure. I offer the wards of our hospital to show the work, and our work will sustain the position of the physicians in Rochester that have resigned. The post-graduate pupils under my tutelage have been trained in the art of healing, and I will guarantee that each one of them can do this work. If this be true, what a pity it is for the professed Homoeopaths of your city to claim anodynes as needed means of relief.

Be sure to make this point emphatic, that I make, viz: I do not select my remedy any differently in curable and incurable cases. I am firmly convinced that a doctor who cannot select medicine closely enough to cure curable cases, should be trusted in no class of cases. The homoeopathic physician does not know that his cases are incurable, and he selects the remedy, and that remedy palliates the sufferings of the patient in incurable cases and cures the patient in curable ones. The physician is a Homoeopath or he is not (Kent 2012).

9.4 Hahnemann's Flexibility

This flexibility highlighted in Kent's work was also a feature of Hahnemann's, as brilliantly revealed by Little in Part 3 Managing the Case.

By the end of the 1830s Hahnemann was using all the levels of potency available from the lowest to the highest but only in medicinal solutions. It is a known fact that he had both Jenichen's and Karsokoff's high potencies. We have in our possession a copy of a letter written by Madame Hahnemann to an American doctor named Breyfogle in which Melanie answers a question about what Hahnemann's views were on potency and dosage in his later life. This is recorded in Haehl's *Samuel Hahnemann, His Life and Works*, Volume 1, on page 328.

"Your inquiry as to whether Hahnemann altered his views about potencies in the last period of life and whether he made use of only high potencies, I can answer in this way: Hahnemann used all the degrees of dilutions, the lower as well as the higher according to the individual case. I have seen him use the 3rd trituration but I have also seen him use 200th and even 1000, every time he thought it necessary."

That fact that Hahnemann used high potencies was confirmed in 1845 in the Bulletin de la Societe Homoepathique de Paris by a Dr. Molin. Also a Dr. Malan witnessed Hahnemann using the latest of Jenichen's ultra high potencies effectively in Paris. This is recorded in Haehl's *Samuel Hahnemann, His Life and Works*, on page 328.

"I frequently saw Hahnemann prescribe very high dilutions. One of the most remarkable cures had been brought about by one single dose of a very high potency: as far as I know this remedy came from Jenichen. I have often heard him say that the 30c potency should by no means form a fixed limit for medicinal dilutions."

It has been said by some modern homoeopaths that Hahnemann never used potencies beyond the 30c. For this reason they opine that his case management suggestion can be ignored when using higher potencies. James Kent made a similar statement in his writings as he was not aware of Hahnemann's use of high potencies and his advanced methods. Once Hahnemann developed the medicinal solutions he found the freedom necessary to experiment with the highest potencies available at the time. The aqueous solution is a perfect medium for controlling the power of the high potencies because the dose can be carefully adjusted to fit the sensitivity of the individual. (Little Hahnemann's Advanced Methods, Part 3 Managing the Case 1996-2007).

More History and Hahnemann's Flexibility

David Little has highlighted how in his later years, in the 1830s, Hahnemann demonstrated extraordinary flexibility in his treatment plans. His client was Duke Valmy, who was unmarried, and was 35 years old. Valmy's case history is suggestive of venereal miasms, suppression, and Mercury poisoning. He visited the good doctor complaining of throat pain, loose teeth, bleeding, pus of the gums, ulcers, and apthae.

These symptoms began after taking a sea journey at the age of 25. His throat pains were treated with bleeding by leeches. Fourteen days before his visit he suffered a relapse of the pain but it passed off naturally. He was constipated and needed to take enemas of water to pass stool. For three years he suffered arthritic pains and edema of the left knee that was worse when fatigued by walking. He was also treated with Mercury for blood of the urethra although the date is not given. Complex diseases involving miasms, suppression, and drug poisoning are the most difficult to cure.

In the 1st edition of *The Chronic Diseases* (1828) the Founder wrote that the treatment of the venereal miasms by allopathic Mercury often causes a flare-up of latent Psora producing an obstructive layer. For this reason he used *Sulphur*, and other anti psoric remedies in many of his suppressed VD cases. By removing the Psora, and the suppression, the VD would then surface unmasked. The Paris casebooks are full of patients with infectious Itch miasm, sycosis, syphilis, and tuberculosis mistreated by the crudest allopathy imaginable. Gay Pari was reeling under the influence of many acute and chronic miasms as well as faulty medical practice. The following is Hahnemann's July 26th prescription.

Sulphur, 1 pill, 30c, in 500 drops of mixture. 1 drop in 6 tablespoons of water. Take one tablespoon every morning.

This is an example of a miniature solution made with 1 pill in 500 drops of 50% brandy and water. After succussing this bottle he placed 1 drop of solution into 6 tablespoons of water in a glass. The water in the glass was then stirred and 1 tablespoon was given to the client as a dose. This technique is called a split dose instead of a multiple dose because it only uses 1 pill to make an aqueous solution that is then 'split' over several days, weeks, or months. In this way, it is possible to take "1 pill many times". This keeps the amount of the dose very small allowing for the repetition of the remedy to speed the cure if and when necessary. He referred to this method in the Paris 1837 edition of *The Chronic Diseases*.

In the year 1837 Hahnemann was still facing several limitations in his therapeutic system, especially in cases like Duke de Valmy. At this time the Founder was working with around 100 remedies in 30c. Although he spoke of potencies above 30c in the 5th *Organon*, in 1837 he mostly used 60c, 30c, 24c, 18c, 12c, and 6c. It is only in 1839 that his journals show him regularly administering the 198c, 199c, or 200c. By 1840 we find him using a full range of C potencies [6c-200c] side by side with his new LM potencies 1/0 to 0/30. The increased remedial powers of the high potency C and LM potency were critical to the development of the complete homoeopathic paradigm.

On September 12th, Valmy was aggravated *Sulphur* 24c in 15 tablespoons of water and given placebo, but he misunderstood the instructions, and continued to take the remedy also. When returning on September 20, Hahnemann gave him *Sulphur* in alternation with a placebo by the symptoms, and on October 23 he gave a series of placebos without *Sulphur*. Valmey's second prescription was given after three months of interspersing placebos with *Sulphur* in various combinations. In this case the good doctor used both the small dropper bottle dose and the larger tablespoon solution.

The Second Prescription

On October 28th, 1837 the case journals noted that Valmy has apthae inside the lip again, bleeding gums, but no pain in the knee, shoulder, or chest muscles. The spots itching on the chest had changed to white discolorations and there were no rushes of blood to the head when getting up. Valmy's case demonstrates chronic miasms, suppression, and Mercury poisoning. At this time, Hahnemann makes his second prescription, and changes his remedy to *Cinnabaris*, the red sulfate of Mercury, a well known anti syphilitic remedy.

R$_x$ *Cinnabaris*, 30c 1 pill in 15 tablespoons with 1 spirit, 1 tablespoon in a glass of water to take 1, 2, 3 increasing small spoons.

In this prescription Hahnemann uses a standard sized medicinal solution that is made in 7 to 15 tablespoons of water [3 1/2 to 7 ounces] with spirits as a preservative. After succussing the remedy bottle, 1 tablespoon was stirred into a glass of water, and 1, 2, 3, or increasingly more teaspoons were given until reaction was attained. This method of using a dilution glass was first published in the 6th edition of the *Organon*, which introduced the LM potency. This case shows that he administered his C potencies exactly like his LM potencies for his last 5 years.

The Founder used the 30c, 24c, 18c, and 6c in their descending order through out his entire career. It is only in the 1840's that we find him raising the potency from 198c to 199c to 200c and using the LM 0/1, 0/2, 0/3 in the ascending order. Nevertheless, he still seemed to favor progressively lowering the degree of his lower potencies 30c to 6c. This opens the C potency scale to an upward or downward movement depending on whether one is using the high or low potencies. The *Cinnabaris* prescription began a series of remedies that started on October 28, 1837 and continued to March 27, 1838. In the last entry Valmy was much better than when he came (Little 1996-2007 Following in Hahnemann's Footsteps. The Definitive Years 1833-1843).

Little's articles on the case books of Hahnemann and his prescribing in the latter years of his life are compulsory reading. One is left with an impression of a balanced, flexible, non-dogmatic prescriber. The posology is varied and the case management patient focussed.

The Homoeopathy of the 1840s

The sixth edition of the *Organon* was completed in 1842 when Hahnemann was 87 years old and is the fruit of his life long experiments. On February 20th, 1842 he wrote a letter to Baron von Bönninghausen to announce the completion of his new work.

"I have now, after 18 months of work finished the sixth edition of my *Organon*, the most nearly perfect of all."

Hahnemann planned for the printing of this final work, but unfortunately, problems arose with his publishers. For this reason, the 6th edition was not published before he died on July 2nd, 1843. It would take more than 80 years before his masterpiece was rescued from obscurity and presented to the homoeopathic community. It is recorded on page 74 of *Boenninghausen's Lesser Writings* that Hahnemann had shared the new LM potency with the Baron.

"In the new edition of the *Organon*, improved and completed by Hahnemann himself, a new simplified procedure for the potentizing of medicine will be taught, which has considerable advantages over the former and yields a preparation as to the efficiency of which I can, from my own experience, give full praise."

Boenninghausen's contribution to homeopathy is vast as he gave us the first complete homeopathic repertories and the relationship of remedies. That the Baron's stated that he was speaking from his "own experience" shows that he had tested the LM remedies. He considered them to have a medicinal power similar to the higher potency Cs rather than a low potency. Hahnemann's low potencies were 30c, 24c, 18c, 12c, 6c and 3c. His high potency range ran from 50c to 200c [tested 1M] and LM 0/1-0/30. He often alternated a placebo with his remedies at various intervals, or followed a series of doses w th placebos. The idea that he used the daily dose for weeks, months, or years in Paris is a complete myth.

The 10 years between the writing of the 5th and 6th *Organon* were the most productive of Samuel Hahnemann's long career. The homeopathy of the 1840's is based on the use of the C and LM remedies in medicinal solution and the repetition of the split dose, when necessary. One of his first LM cases was started in 1840 with *Sulphur* 0/10 causing a strong aggravation that was treated with placebos for some time. In the beginning, he tried to move downward from 0/10, 0/9, 0/8 as he had done with his lower potency Cs. He soon found that the new LM remedies were high potencies and then changed to starting in the lowest degrees like 0/1, 0/2, 0/3, and then moving upward through the scale. By the year 1843 he began most of his LM cases between 0/1 and 0/3, although occasionally he would start at 0/4, 0/5, 0/6, etc., depending on the circumstances.

The following is a redaction of a Paris case dated January 14th, 1843, just six months before Hahnemann left for his Heavenly Abode. On this client he used the C and LM potencies in medicinal solution at different times in the case. This example was sent by letter to Boenninghausen and is recorded on page 192 of the Baron's Lesser Writings.

"O-t, an actor, 33 years old, married. 14 January, 1843. For several years he had been frequently subject to sore throats as also now for a month past. The previous sore throat had lasted six weeks. On swallowing his saliva, a pricking sensation, feeling of contraction and excoriation. When he does not have the sore throat he suffers from a pressure in the anus, with violent excoriated pains, the anus is then inflamed swollen and constricted; it is only with great effort that he can pass his stool, then the swollen hemorrhoidal vessels protrude."

On January 15th Hahnemann gave 1 pill of *Belladonna 30c* in a 7-tablespoon medicinal solution that was succussed just prior to administration. One tablespoon was then taken and stirred in a glass of water. The exact number of succussions and the dosage given to the patient is not noted. By the next day, the sore throat was gone, but the old rectal affection had resurfaced as an anal fissure. Under questioning the actor confessed that he had contracted syphilis eight years earlier that was treated with caustics. This confirmed that the doctor was treating a case of active secondary syphilis. He then administered *Belladonna's* anti syphilitic complement *Merc. Viv. LM 0/1.*

"*Merc. Viv.* one globule of the lowest new dynamization. (which contains a vastly smaller amount of matter than the usual kind), prepared in the same manner, and to be taken in the same as the *Belladonna* (the bottle being shaken each time), one spoonful in a tumblerful of water well stirred."

The Founder then repeated the dose of *Merc* LM 0/1 and LM 0/2 until January 30th when the throat became inflamed again. He then used a placebo for seven days until February 7th. By then the anus was better but the sore throat was still lingering. He then realized that Psora was interfering with his anti-syphilitic remedy as he warned about such things in the Chronic Diseases. Hahnemann then used his cardinal anti-psoric remedy, *Sulphur* in LM 0/2 as a chronic intercurrent, and repeated the dose until February 13th.

During this period the client developed clear Mercury symptoms like ulcerative pains in the throat and profuse saliva, so on Feburary 13th he was again given *Merc. Viv.*, LM 0/2. The Sulphur had removed the obstructive layer of Psora and suppression allowing the syphilitic symptoms to surface. By the 20th the sore throat was completely gone and the anus once again became inflamed and hemorrhoidal. The Founder now used placebo for 13 days! Hahnemann favored the alternate day over the daily dose and often interpolated placebos with his remedies. His case journals put an end to the myth that he used the daily dose for weeks, months and years on end.

On the 3rd of March the sore throat was gone, but the patient experienced blind piles that protruded at stool, but the pains were much better. Hahnemann then prescribed *Nitric Acid* by olfaction [potency unknown]. The patient was given milk sugar in medicinal solution as a placebo to keep him under control. According to the Founder's notes, "He remained perfectly cured". After first giving *Belladonna 30c* as an acute remedy, Hahnemann used 3 anti-miasmatic remedies in 3 months, *Merc viv.*, *Sulphur*, and *Nitric Acid*.

A letter of Dr. Croserio's, Hahnemann's close colleague in his 3 last years, states that he never saw Hahnemann alternate remedies. If one investigates the Paris case journals very closely an occasional alternation is noted under special circumstances. In the LM period [1840-1843] such prescriptions are indeed so rare that Croserio did not even notice them in his visits. One interesting example of alternation is the case of *Madam Gardy, 44 years old, who was seen on April 18, 1842.

Madam Gardy suffered from womb problems since a childbirth 19 years prior that was treated with a variety of suppressive treatments. This complex chronic state was then complicated by a crisis caused by cerebral fevers. Hahnemann began this case with an alternation of *Aconite 30c* and *Sulphur* LM 0/5 in medicinal solution. The case improved radically and the crisis was overcome. We note these unusual cases in which he used alternations, or an intercurrent remedy to complement his constitutional treatment. This is an alternation of two remedies as well as the C and LM potency systems. In this way, any promising techniques may be tested in clinical trials and updated if found effective. (*A case from the author's collection of microfiches obtained from the Robert Bosch Institute, Germany).

The higher and highest potencies (200c, 1M, 10M, and above) must be used with great caution in cases where there are special sensitivities or too much tissue pathology. Therefore, in many serious diseases there is very little leeway in the choice of potency. Sometimes the lower C potencies are not deep enough to cure while the higher C potencies only produce unproductive aggravations. This is one of the times the LM potency may be a lifesaver. When the C potencies are used in the split-dose of the medicinal solutions they act more like the LM potencies yet each pharmaceutical method retains its individual character.

It may be noted in the Paris casebooks that Hahnemann used his Cs in crisis and acute conditions, and his LMs for chronic degenerative disorders and chronic miasms. This tendency, however, was neither absolute nor exclusive as he sometimes used the Cs in chronic cases, and the LM in acutes. The C and LM potencies in medicinal solution greatly expanded the therapeutic horizons of classical homoeopathy when compared with the 4th *Organon* techniques and the dry dose.

Samuel Hahnemann worked for 50 years to perfect his new healing art. The final definitive years were 1840 to 1843, the epoch around the creation of the 6th *Organon*. Unfortunately, the Paris period is being misrepresented by a number of so-called reformers of our healing art. They speak as if the Paris casebooks contain some new revelation that sweeps away the cardinal principles of homoeopathy. They use polypharmacy terms like "dual remedies" and "combinations" to describe the Founder's use of alternation and a series of remedies. "Hahnemann, Hahnemann, Hahnemann" they cry while in truth they use too many remedies or mixtures chosen by so-called causations or disease names. This has confused new students as well as old practitioners that are only familiar with the methods of the 4th *Organon*. Their hubris knows no bounds.

The 1840-1843 Paris casebooks, and the 6th edition of the *Organon of the Healing Art*, contain the seeds of the best of contemporary homoeopathy, and much more. Those trained in the 4th *Organon* and the wait and watch method are the best prepared to test the hypothesis of the Paris methods in the clinic. Without this solid foundation in homoeopathy it is almost impossible to understand the sophisticated posology techniques, and case management procedures of the 1840's. Why allow our heritage to be misrepresented and abused by the pretenders? Hahnemann's advanced methods require more knowledge of classical methods not less. Homoeopaths, Dare to know! (Little 1996-2007 Following in Hahnemann's Footsteps. The Definitive Years 1833-1843).

What makes David Little's work so important is the way he has meticulously charted and mapped the origins of case management from the start. This is not to say that because Hahnemann did this, we should all or always follow. But rather to my mind, it highlights that when we have accurate information about the origins of the profession then we can make balanced and reasons suggestions. This is different from guesswork and simply making it up. Little's description of the correct interpretation and action following a prescription, the different types of aggravation, the way in which Hahnemann developed methods to adjust the dose of the remedy to fit the sensitivity of the constitution of the patient, are again important reading. In the important article Hahnemann's Advanced Methods, Part Three, Managing the Case, Little charts went to repeat, when the remedy is wrong, and how to follow a case to completion. He gives excellent examples using some centessimal and 50 milessimal potencies and above all, how to complete the cure.

When it comes to the sixth edition of the *Organon* Little provides the history of the development of the fifth and sixth editions and the differences in various paragraphs between the two books. He then gives an excellent contemporary example.

An Example of a LM Single Dose Cure

While working in the hill district of Himachal Pradesh, in North India a teenage girl was presented to me with the following symptoms: Her left foot and lower leg had been terribly infected for at least a year and now there was advanced blood poisoning and a danger of gangrene. She had been given antibiotics several times but they did not help her.

Her foot and lower leg were very cold and there was numbness, tingling, burning, itching, swelling and an angry red blister-like eruption. The veins of her legs were swollen and icy cold and the condition was aggravated in the cold weather or when the cold wind blew down out of the mountains. These symptoms represented the location, sensations, and modifications of the chief complaint.

I now began to probe for some concomitants to fill out the case. Most people with such a serious complaint are very anxious or afraid yet she bore her suffering bravely. I asked her how she did in school and she mentioned to me that she had trouble reading because the letters seemed to move or appear double. This would give her headaches and make it hard to study. As her eye condition had nothing to do with her chief complaint I looked up this concomitant in the repertory immediately. Under Vision; moving; letters; I found *Agar, am-c., con., Hyos., iod., merc., phys.*.

Then it struck me! Her leg looked and felt like it had been **frozen**. I quickly looked up Fearlessness because she seemed so brave under the condition she faced and found, *Agar., bell., coca., OP., sil.*. The coldness of the limb, the numbness, tingling, the blistered eruptions are all found in the materia medica under the remedy *Agaricus*. Agaricus LM 0/1 was made in a 6 oz. remedy solution and the patient was given one teaspoon as a dose and told to return the next day.

The next day the foot and leg looked much better! The swelling was down and the girl seemed happy. I did not repeat the dose because this response was "striking." I told her to come back in three days if the leg continued to improve but immediately if there was any relapse. She came back in three days and the leg was looking much better. The blisters were healing, the red diminishing, and the blood poisoning was reduced. I told her to come back in one week. After a week she returned walking on her foot. It looked so much better it was amazing.

I told her to come back once a week unless there was a relapse of the symptoms. The next week her foot was completely healed and warm. All of this took place in just under three weeks. This is an example of a single dose of an LM 0/1 causing a "striking rapid cure". A single dose of LM 0/1 is not to be underestimated. One dose of a LM 0/1 has removed severe attacks of asthma for 9 months before a relapse. A few more doses and the case was cleared. We have seen this type of response many times.

When using the LM potency it is always best to give a single dose and ask the patient to come back in 3 to 7 days, or more, depending on the nature of the disease. Cases of slowly developing chronic diseases may take a little longer to clearly show the reaction to the first dose. If the patient has a "striking" reaction to the remedy the repetition of the dose is contraindicated. If the dramatic healing reaction slows down the time has come to examine the case to see if it is time for the second dose. The remedy should then be repeated to see how it acts the second time. One may find that an infrequent repetition of the remedy is all that is necessary.

If the reaction is not very dramatic then the remedy may be introduced at intervals that correspond to the reaction of the constitution. The LM potency should not be repeated mechanically as if they are a 6x remedy! The LM system is far too deep acting for this kind of approach and demands sensitivity and flexibility in the homoeopath's hands. The wait and watch philosophy is still a very important part of Hahnemann's advanced methods.

In addition, Little's article, Speeding the Cure is a gem. Exploring different clinical situations, it provides grounded advice on what to do when the first dose acts, when it is slow to act, when there is a striking amelioration during treatment, or slow progressive improvement. He argues that speeding the cure, more doses in a slow moving case, is permissible when the remedy is homeopathic, when the remedy is potentised, in liquid and given in the appropriate dose, in clearly defined intervals of repetition, and ensuring that each dose is different through succussion (Little 1996-2007 Hahnemann's Advanced Methods. Part five: Speeding the Cure).

9.5 Little's Best Practice

The amount of variables in homeopathic prescribing can make it bewildering for new practitioners. There are so many pieces of advice, often conflicting, and often with their own justifications. What I have attempted to do here is provide the landscape for the variations. From Hahnemann through to Kent, Close, Roberts, Henriques to de Schepper. Individual homeopaths will have their own variations and nuances also. In his article, Refining the Paradigm (1996-2007) David Little provides the context and reasons for his decision-making process in a contemporary practice. There are minor adjustments from Hahnemann's directives. They are all resoned excellently. The daily dose is not always used. Neither is the single dose. Flexibility is the most obvious feature but it is the reasoned process behind it that makes it such important reading.

1. **I begin my cases with a single test dose (C or LM) of a well chosen remedy, potency, and dose adjustments.** Under rare circumstances I may give a short series of three test doses at the most suitable intervals (daily, alternate day, every three days, every four days, etc.). In this case, I tell the patient to stop the medicine immediately if there is any aggravation, new symptoms or a strikingly progressive improvement. I only do this with relatively hyposensitive patients with stable vitality that live too far away for me to observe the

case more closely in the beginning. In India most people do not have a phone.

2. **When there is a strikingly progressive amelioration from a single test dose, or a short series of test doses, the remedy is not repeated.** This is because there is no need to speed the cure. My colleagues and I have witnessed many cases cured by a single dose and infrequent repetitions.

   A. **Once the strikingly progressive amelioration slows down the remedy may be repeated at similar intervals to continue the rapid cure.** If the strikingly progressive amelioration last for 3, 4, 5, or 6 days, I repeat the remedy every 3, 4, 5, or 6 days. If the progressive improvement last for 1, 2, 3, or 4 weeks, I give the remedy every 1, 2, 3, or 4 weeks. If the progressive improvement lasts for 1, 2, 3, 4 months, I give the remedy every 1, 2, 3, or 4 months, etc. If it lasts for 1, 2, 3 or 4 years I give the remedy every 1, 2, 3 or 4 years, etc.

3. **When there is little or no amelioration or only a slow improvement in response to the single test dose, or short series of test doses, the remedy is repeated at more rapid intervals.** These suitable intervals are (as Hahnemann said) what "experience has shown to be the most suitably appropriate for the best possible acceleration of the cure".

   A. I judge the appropriate intervals in accordance with the sensitivity of the patient, the nature and stage of the disease state, the age of the patient, and the state of their vitality. Those that seem hyposensitive yet have relatively stable vitality may receive the remedy daily. Those that seem a little less hyposensitive may receive the remedy on alternate days. Those that are a little more sensitive may receive the remedy every three or four days, etc. At this time the patient is given a series of three to seven doses to see if the sensitivity and disease condition has been judged correctly. **I tell the patient to stop the remedy immediately if there is any aggravation, new symptoms, or strikingly progressive amelioration.**

B. If the chosen interval produces a satisfactory improvement the remedy is continued at this rhythm to speed the cure. **When the patient experiences a significant improvement these intervals are slowed because the patient no longer needs as much medicinal stimulation.** In this way aggravations in the middle of treatment can be avoided.

C. **When the patient reaches the point where they no longer show any symptoms, and the vitality has completely returned, the medicine is stopped to test the cure.** If there is no relapse of symptoms after waiting and watching for a reasonable amount of time they are cured. If some of the symptoms return the remedy is again repeated at slightly longer intervals to complete the cure.

D. **If there is an aggravation toward the end of treatment the medicine is stopped and a period of waiting and watching is begun.** If the symptoms pass off quickly, and the patient does not relapse, the cure is complete. When there is a return of symptoms the remedy is again administered but at slightly longer intervals in order to prevent any reoccurrence of the aggravation and complete the cure. After carrying out this procedure the methods described in point 3C or point 3D are repeated if necessary (Little, Refining the Paradigm 1996-2007).

9.6 Lippe

In this context, the last word goes to Lippe, arguably one of the greatest ever prescribers of homeopathy.

The question of doses has been discussed for a long time, and many are the arguments and reasonings offered in the medical journals of our school; but the question is not any nearer a satisfactory solution than when it was first started the paper which I have the privilege of reading before my colleagues today proposes to show the reasons why this question has not been solved—why it cannot yet be solved and must remain an open question till the solution is made practicable by means not yet at our command.

In order to do this, let us first take a retrospective, historical view of this question of doses; dwell for a moment upon its present position; point out the reasons why the solution is an impossibility at present; indicate the preliminary steps which must be taken in order to enable us to come to a final conclusion; and, finally, show how we have to proceed to take these steps and so present the question as to make its solution a possibility.

When Hahnemann first established the correctness of the Homoeopathic law of cure, the law of similars, be employed in his first experimental trials crude medicines in comparatively very small doses, smaller than the common school of medicine were in the habit of prescribing; but he found these comparatively small doses, when applied in accordance with the law of similars, caused such violent aggravation of sufferings that he was compelled to seek for means to avoid this great difficulty, and for that reason only did he resort, at first, to what he then called "dilutions," or rather a mere division of quantities. At a later period, while proving *Carbo vegetabilis*, he illustrated, by the practical experiment to his followers, the theory of potentiation for the first time. The crude charcoal produced no effects on the provers, and then Hahnemann showed his pupils how to develop medicinal powers out of an otherwise inert substance, by trituration. And when the provers began to be affected by potencies of a substance which, in its crude state, had not developed any change of sensation in them, they became convinced of Hahnemann's correct observations; and their conviction grew stronger in degree as they further found that symptoms obtained by them from the potentized charcoal were true and reliable guides, under the law of the similars, in the selection of that remedy for the cure of the sick. Hahnemann found further, by experiment, that all other medicinal substances gained curative powers by potentiation; caused fewer aggravations of already existing symptoms, and were more efficacious in curing the sick. Hahnemann gradually diminished the dose, and this diminution kept pace with his increasing knowledge of the medicinal power of drugs by proving them, and by administering them to the sick, guided by the law of cure and the provings. And when Hahnemann published the *Chronic Diseases*, be declared that we will find the thirtieth potency all-sufficient, provided the symptoms of the remedy correspond with those of the disease, or in other words, if the remedy is truly Homoeopathic to the case.

And even at that time there were found among his pretended followers men like Griesslich, who not only stubbornly refused to accept the small doses, but bitterly assailed the master on that account; and even then began the question of expediency against principle. This faction was wholly discarded by Hahnemann, and the most charitable construction we can possibly put on their conduct is this, that they imagined Homoeopathy, as a new school, would be more acceptable to the Allopaths if it could only come before them without the so objectionable and so ridiculous pellet.

Hahnemann was not the man to yield to expediencies; he continued to diminish the doses, and all the opposition and slanders could not check him, and his fame increased day by day. His cures became a greater certainty as he advanced in knowledge and as he decreased the doses; and we are informed by reliable persons that the last edition of the *Organon*, which Madam Hahnemann has for some time contemplated publishing, from his MS. in her possession, will show that he came to give still smaller doses than the thirtieth, as he advanced in experience. During Hahnemann's time do we find Korsacoff carrying the potencies much higher than before; and later, Jenichen proposed to potentize medicines till he reached a point at which they would no longer retain curative qualities. He did this with fear and trembling, and the experiments made by him on himself, and by a few friends on themselves and others, revealed only the fact, that these, by him so called high-potencies not only retained their curative powers, but that diseased conditions were cured by them when lower potencies had produced no beneficial effects.

In our days, we find our colleague, Dr. Fincke, following up the experiment; and he has carried the potencies to a much higher degree than any one before him. And we are assured by the testimony of such physicians as have carefully tried them, that they not only cured patients, but it is asserted that they are by far the most curative agents ever employed. Not only have they been serviceable as curative agents, but the very highest potencies have been proved on the healthy, and the results obtained show the reliability of the experimental provings.

The opposition, which Griesslich & Co. began, (against the smaller doses) has continued ever since, and, while he and those who followed him made it a question of expediency, we find others governed by principles only. Admitting the honesty of purpose of all contending parties, their object being to advance our school, it is obvious to the close observer of history, that expediencies never accomplish what can only be obtained by a strict adherence to principles. The belief of honest and well meaning physicians that the common school of medicine will adopt Homoeopathy, if we only give up the theory of potentiation, is a grave error.

Again, we find, on the one side, those who are governed by the question of expediency not only give up one of the great principles, that of potentiation, but more or less other principles and most of the practical rules taught by Hahnemann. And, on the other side, we find those who have faithfully carried out the practical rules of Hahnemann, and are governed strictly by the principles taught by him, adhering to the smaller doses. On the one side, the small doses are entirely rejected; and on the other side, the question of doses is left open to the choice of the physician in each individual case. As a general thing, these latter prefer the higher potentized medicine, but hold that we have not yet found the law which must govern us in the selection of the dose in each individual case. And, while contending for the "minimum dose,"that is, the dose just sufficient to cure, they admit that it must still remain an open question, what that minimum dose is in each individual case.

The question of doses was generally understood to be the question whether larger or smaller doses, lower or higher potencies, were more preferable and more successful in the cure of the sick. And the very fact of asking such a question, implied the supposition that either the lower or higher potencies were more efficacious in all cases, and that we were striving to generalize one way or the other. But since such a generalizing solution of the question is outside of, and incompatible with, the avowed Homoeopathic principles of "individualizing,"the question so put never was satisfactorily answered, and never will be. The reflecting mind will seek a solution by a different mode of investigation. If we acknowledge the law of the similars as a fundamental principle in Homoeopathy, we must apply that law in the selection of the remedy for the cure of the sick, and individualize in each and every case. Under the guidance of this principle, we cannot possibly expect to find specific medicines for specific forms of dis-eases; and—which is the same thing—we cannot generalize. To be more explicit, we find that *Belladonna* is not a specific for scarlet fever, nor *Pulsatilla* for measles, nor *China* for intermittent fever; since our avowed principle compels us to individualize in the selection of the truly curative medicine in each and every case. And, if we admit this, does it not follow, as a logical conclusion, that we must likewise find in each individual case the true minimum dose for that case? that we can as little generalize in the selection of the dose as we could in the selection of the remedy ?

And we must so much the more become convinced of the fruitlessness of the means hitherto resorted to, to solve a question which was not rightly put, if we look but for a moment at the unsatisfactory results obtained. To sustain this proposition, it is not necessary to dwell at length on the various articles published on the subject, for or against; the exclusive use of either the lower or higher potencies; they have not brought the question nearer solution, for the obvious reasons above shown.

And we only refer here to the experimental trials of doses as reported by Dr. Eidberr, in Vienna. These trials were made during ten consecutive years, from 1650 to 1660. All cases of pneumonia occurring in the Leopoldstadt Hospital, at Vienna, were treated for the first three years with the 80th potency; for the second period of three years with the 6th potency; and for the last four years with the 15th potency. The average time of sickness during the first three years, under the 30th potency, was 11.3 days: during the second three years, with the 6th potency, it was 19.5 days; during the third period of four years, under the 15th dilution, it was 14.6 days; showing conclusively that the results were in favor of the higher potencies and that, in the same ratio as the medicines were administered in higher potencies, the duration of the disease became shorter. And even this very elaborate report proved but little; the only deduction which can possibly be drawn from it is, that the higher potencies proved to be superior to the lower ones in the treatment of one acute disease. The report has met the same fate as did the relation of other scattered facts on record, showing that in some isolated cases the higher potencies bad been applied with great success. The adherents to the larger doses and opponents of dynamization ignored these reports, taking no notice of them, and, in some instances, they (vide Pope's articles) unhesitatingly acknowledged their utter ignorance of the existence of the elaborate report above referred to, or of other similar facts published in the journals.

And, from the consideration of all these facts, it is apparent that the question of doses remains an open one at present; it must be left to the choice of the physician to select, in each individual case, the dose according to the best of his own judgment, and that the whole range of doses must be left open to his choice. And this is the doctrine of doses taught in the Homoeopathic Medical College of Pennsylvania for the last three years,—all the assertions to the contrary notwithstanding. It is true that, in the Dispensary and Public Clinic connected with this College, the patients have been exclusively treated with the higher and highest potencies. The results of this treatment will be laid before the profession. The journals are carefully kept by members of the class, and it will be an easy task to make an extract from them, and give a report, not with the intention of settling definitely the question of doses: far from it: the report can only show whether the higher and highest potencies are capable of curing diseased conditions, and in what time and to what extent, and it can show nothing more. The investigating physicians will be free to draw such deductions and conclusions from comparisons of this with other reports as the facts may warrant.

If it is admitted that the question of doses remains for the present an open one, that the modes of investigating it have not brought it to a solution, because they were all in themselves in opposition to the avowed principle of individualization, it follows, therefore, that another mode of investigating the question must be pursued. And it is now my object to propose a plan which may lead to this end. And if you will only follow me in my reasoning before adapting or rejecting the proposed plan, I hope you will accept it as the only feasible means of solving the question at issue.

When we wish to apply the law of similars to the cure of the sick, we seek for the truly Homoeopathic remedy in our Materia Medica; and the same great repository of the knowledge of drug-action may also be applied to for the solution of the vexed question of the dose. Our Materia Medica is composed of, and has been obtained by, provings of medicines on the human organism; these provings have been made with large crude doses and with various potencies; different provers with differing individualities, of different sexes, ages, and temperaments, at different times and in different localities, under varying circumstances, have responded similarly, but differently to different and various doses. So-called diseases also cause variously differing symptoms on different individuals, endowed with differing individualities, and their effects on each person are modified by the same conditions as are the effects of medicines on the provers. For instance, miasm and contagion will affect different individuals, either not at all, or similarly but differently: the altered conditions in both instances are modified by the individuality of the subject exposed to either of them, that is, the medicine or the disease. If these propositions are correct, we can and must draw the conclusion from them, that we can neither find a specific for a disease nor a uniform dose for every person suffering from the influence of disease; that in either case we must individualize and not generalize. If these propositions and the conclusions drawn from them are correct, they also carry with them the means of solving the question of doses. In order to solve this question, we must know—

1. What symptoms composing our Materia Medica were observed from crude drugs, what from the lower, the higher, and the highest potencies.

2. What symptoms were observed from all of them, and what symptoms only from the one or the other preparation.

3. Do the symptoms observed from all of them yield to all doses, or do they yield sooner or more permanently to the one or the other dose, and to which dose do they most readily yield?

4. Do the symptoms observed from large doses yield to the higher potencies?

5. Do the symptoms observed from higher potencies yield to lower potencies?

6. Do higher potencies cure cases which did not improve under lower potencies, or vice versa?

7. Must we ascend or descend in the scale of potencies, if the remedy has been truly Homoeopathic to the case, and if the dose administered did not cause any improvement?

In a small way, we might, even at present, make an effort to have these questions answered, as we are in the possession of provings with *Apis, Sulphur, Thuya, Lachesis, Camphor, Lachnanthes, Gelseminum*, in all known doses, and with such remedies as *Theridion*, only proved in the 30th potency. But in order to arrive at a satisfactory solution of all these questions, we must be in the possession of a complete Materia Medica, and if the results of the experiment have solved the proposed questions, we will be in the possession of such facts as will enable us to draw conclusions from them, and they again will further serve as an unerring guide in the selection of the similar dose in every individual case. Till we have a Materia Medica, as above indicated, the question of doses must remain an open one, and be left, as it always has been, to the judgment of the practitioner in each individual case.

And, if the above arguments are admitted, it becomes also obvious that, as Homoeopathicians, we cannot admit a distinction, which persons who deny the efficacy and admissibility of higher potencies contrary to historical facts, have been diligently endeavoring to make,— I mean the distinguishing and division of members of our school into high and low potency men. All honest men will no doubt join me in the desire and aid in the effort to solve the pending question; and till it is solved, till we have obtained practical rules derived from the experiments to be instituted, we must stand united and aid one another in this great work.

To show, in a familiar way, the utter absurdity of dividing our school into high and low potency men, you will please allow me to draw a timely comparison. And, for the present, I will only compare those so-called Homoeopathicians who totally reject and deny the efficacy of high potencies, and thereby wish to create a sect of their own and discredit those who admit the high potencies as logical consequence of the fundamental principles of Homoeopathy with those of our fellow-citizens who, although living in the Republic and pretending to be members of the large body politic, deny the principle of equal rights and of manhood Suffrage as a logical consequence of the fundamental laws of our institutions.

And, in the lapse of time, I trust we shall hear the last of the silly pretence that we must drop a logical conclusion because the pellet will stink in the nostrils of our enemies—the common school of medicine—a school which carries within itself the germs of its own destruction, because not founded, as is ours, on the laws of nature—a school without any principles at all, guided solely by expediencies, will be laughed to scorn; such pretences will avail as little as do the waitings of interested slave-drivers and enemies of the republic, who contend that equal rights and manhood suffrage would be offensive to the delicate nostrils of crowned heads abroad and to the tender sensibilities of an aping aristocracy at home!

The logical consequences must come. In the one instance they are already come; in the other they must come also. And may I be spared the distasteful duty to follow my argument out according to strictly logical principles, to show what unenviable position the blind adherents to expediency must necessarily occupy, as long, as a position is left them at all, which can be but a short time. And if this paper, which you have heard me read tonight, can persuade reflecting, honest men to discuss the question at issue impassionately, guided by facts and logic, I shall consider its preparation one of the happiest events of my life (Lippe A 1867).

Conclusion Case Management

This book has focused on understanding where we come from. Because case management is so critical to success in practice, we do need to identify the origins of what we do. That is why this book explores in significant depth the writings and the literature from the old masters to the present day. The views of different authors have been presented without favour. Proponents of the fourth edition of the *Organon*, sit alongside authors advocating prescribing according to the fifth or sixth edition of the *Organon of Medicine*. It is important that we make our own minds up. Clarity comes from potentisation, and in this context that means reading and learning on the one hand and the coal face of practice on the other. Ultimately each practitioner must come to a comfortable place where they are able to maximize their understanding and skills, with the type of practice they have, above all always seeking the best results for the clients.

In presenting the material in this way, it is been my sincere wish that each individual homeopath understands the lineage, not to necessarily persuade them to change their views or the minds or even do something different, but to understand more deeply the context of why they do what they doing. After twenty years teaching undergraduates in the classroom, case management is, along with miasmatic theory, the area of homeopathic practice where students struggle the most and seek answers and clarity. There can only be principles and suggestions but not laws in this regard. Psychotherapists have developed different models to assist with their case management work. Some, like the Egan model (2009), can be very useful, especially in knowing at which point a patient is at in their process. Homeopathy is still in it's infancy in having this kind of structure.

Now with the underpinnings and the traditions of case management in homeopathy established, we can turn our attention to the practical application of these principles in the consulting room. Learning homeopathy has got very little in common with being a homeopath. The subsequent volume to this work will focus on complex, difficult, and complicated patient management in contemporary contexts. The next book grounds the theory and we explore the messy, visceral, pragmatic and rewarding realities of practice. This next book came out of a number of lectures, webinars, seminars and presentations looking at the history the theory and philosophy working with people living contemporary lifestyles. Anxiety and recreational drug use, along with medical drug addiction and compulsion was seen as the major reasons for rethinking what we have traditionally done in homeopathy. In doing so, I've attempted to set the scene and delineate the reasons for looking at 21st-century patients. It's not easy using gentle medicine in a crazy world. It's busy, fast and dynamic. Further, in traditional or classical homoeopathy we can do have strong values and opinions. And to do what we do and provide the type of healthcare we want, we also need a certain type of information and compliance from our patients. But the reality is that we have to remember that patients have their own ideas about chocolate, salt, smoking, and drugs. Until recently there is been a clear gap between the theory and the pragmatic reality of practice. In this next book I've attempted to identify how to engage with clients, a method moving forward, harm minimisation techniques and strong clinical principles. It's good to remember that a number of these ideas come from working in the western world and a very specific type of practice, and these assumptions and realities may not hold true for every homeopath working in Iceland, India or Brazil.

It will only continue to change. With Gen-X, Gen-Y and now Millenials, patient attitudes to food and lifestyle are a never ending feast of change. Not to mention sex, morality and standards of behaviour. We need to be mindful of the physiological effects of ecstasy, speed, crystal-meth, dope, and mushrooms. 21st-century clients live in a chaotic world. The social media phenomena can only be understood as a generation of people desperate to connect. People obsessed and addicted to Twitter, Facebook, or any other type of social media are desperately seeking connection. In this, they are no different from any other generation that are seeking to engage or connect. The capacity to engage meaningfully with a client is now more than ever fundamental to the practice of homeopathy, not as an excuse for poor prescribing, but because of clients incapacity to give us strong clear characteristic symptoms. As a consequence homeopaths must maximise themselves in the therapeutic equation. It is to that adventure that we now turn.

References

Ayer, A.J. (1956) *The Problem of Knowledge*, Penguin Books, Edinburgh.

Banerjee, P.N. (1984) *Chronic Disease, its cause and cure*, Pratap Medical Publishers Pvt. Ltd. New Delhi.

Banerji, P. (1988) *Advanced Homoeopathy and its Materia Medica* - Volumes I & II, Advanced Thinkers, Calcutta.

Banerjee, P.N. (1984) *The Second Prescription*, accessed in RadarOpus January 2013

Bradford, T.L. (1895) *The Life and Letters of Dr. Samuel Hahnemann*, Roy Publishing House: Calcutta, accessed in RadarOpus 2013.

Burnett, J. (1888) *Fifty Reasons for Being a Homeopath*, accessed in RadarOpus 2013.

Chatterjee, T. P. *Fundamentals of Homoeopathy and Valuable Hints for Practice*, accessed in RadarOpus 2013.

Choudhury, H. 50 *Millesimal Potency in Theory & Practice*, New Delhi: B. Jain Publishers, 1986. 2nd ed., accessed in RadarOpus 2013.

Close, S. (1924) *The Genius of Homeopathy – Lectures and Essays on Homeopathic Philosophy*, B. Jain, New Delhi.

Das, A.K. (1998) *A Treatise on Organon of Medicine*, Calcutta.

De Schepper, L. (2004) *Achieving and Maintaining the Simillimum*, Full of Life Publishing, Sante Fe.

De Schepper, L. (1999) *Hahnemann Revisited: Hahnemannian Textbook of Classical Homeopathy for the Professional*, Full of Life Publishing, Santa Fe.

Dhawale, M. (1967) *Principles & Practice of Homoeopathy*, accessed in RadarOpus 2013.

Dimitriadis, G. (2004) *Homœopathic Diagnosis - Hahnemann through Bönninghausen*. Hahnemann Institute, Sydney.

Egan, G. Ninth International Edition, (2009) *The Skilled Helper*, Wadsworth Publishing Co Inc.

Feldman, R. (2003) *Epistemology*, Prentice Hall.

Freshwater, D. and Rolfe, G. (2004) *Deconstructing Evidence Based Practice*, Routledge

Gamble, J. (2005) *Mastering Homeopathy*, Karuna Publishing, Australia.

Gray, A. (2010) *Case Taking*, The Landscape of Homeopathic Medicine Vol I, BJain/Archibel Assesse, Belgium

Gray, B. (2012) http://www.billgrayhomeopathy.com/interferences/, last accessed Oct 2013.

Gunavante, S.M. *Introduction to Homœopathic Prescribing Management of the Case*, accessed in RadarOpus 2013.

Gunavante, S.M. (1994) *The "Genius" of Homoeopathic Remedies*, B. Jain Publisher (P) Ltd. New Delhi.

Haehl, R. (2006) *Samuel Hahnemann His Life and Work*, Reprint edn., B. Jain Publishers (P) Ltd., New Delhi.

Hahnemann, S. (1921) *Organon of Medicine*, 5th & 6th edn. combined, reprinted 2005, B. Jain Publishers (P) Ltd., New Delhi.

Hahnemann, S. *Organon Of Medicine*, 6th Edition translated by Boericke. http://www.homeopathyhome.com/reference/organon/organon.html. Last accessed Oct 2013.

Hahnemann, S. *The Chronic Diseases, their Peculiar Nature and their Homœopathic Cure*, Presented By Médi-T, http://homeoint.org/books/hahchrdi/hahchr00.htm#P7. Last accessed Oct 2013.

Hahnemann, S. (1896) *The Chronic Diseases, their Peculiar Nature and Homoeopathic Treatment*. Tafel, Louis H, trans. Boericke & Tafel, Philadelphia PA

Henriques, N. (1998) *Crossroads to Cure; the Homoeopath's Guide to the Second Prescription*, Totality Press, St Helena, CA.

Heudens-mast, H. 1998. *An Interview With Henny Heudens-Mast, American Homoeopath*, accessed in RadarOpus 2013.

Hussey, E.P. (1912) *The second prescription*, accessed in RadarOpus 2012.

International Hahnemannian Association 1888, accessed in RadarOpus 2013

Johnston, L. (2012) http://www.homeopathy-md.com/General_Information.html. Last accessed Oct 2013

Jütte, R. (2008) *The doctor-patient relationship as reflected in the case books of Samuel Hahnemann* [online] Hpathy last accessed 16 March 2013 at http://hpathy.com/homeopathy-papers/the-doctor%E2%80%93patient-relationship-as-reflected-in-the-case-books-of-samuel-hahnemann/

Jütte, R. (2005) *Samuel Hahnemann. Begründer der Homöopathie*, Deutsche Taschenbuch Verlag, Munich.

References

Kaplan, B. (2001) *The Homeopathic Conversation: The Art of Taking the Case*, Natural Medicine Press.

Kent, J.T. (1888) *International Hahnemannian Association*, accessed in RadarOpus 2013.

Kent, J.T. (1921) *The Second Prescription* in *Lesser Writings*, accessed in RadarOpus 2013.

Kent, J.T. (1900) *Lectures on Homeopathic Philosophy*, B. Jain Publishers (P) Ltd., New Delhi.

Kent, J.T. (1921) *What the people should know* in *Lesser Writings*, accessed in RadarOpus 2013.

Kent, J.T. (2012) *New Remedies, clinical cases, lesser writings, aphorisms and precepts*, accessed in RadarOpus 2013.

Koehler (1986) *The Handbook of Homoeopathy*, accessed in RadarOpus 2013

Lippe, A. *The Question of Doses/Potentization* Hahnemannian Monthly Dec. 1867, accessed in RadarOpus 2013.

Little, D. 1996-2007 *Following in Hahnemann's Footsteps. The Definitive Years 1833-1843*. http://www.simillimum.com/education/little-library. Last accessed July 2013

Little, D. 1996-2007 *Hahnemann's Advanced Methods. Part five: Speeding the Cure*. http://www.simillimum.com/education/little-library. Last accessed July 2013

Little, D. *Hahnemann's Advanced Methods, Part 3 Managing the Case 1996-2007*. http://www.simillimum.com/education/little-library. Last accessed July 2013

Little, D. *1996-2007 Hahnemann's Advanced Methods Part 1: Hahnemannian Homoeopathy* http://www.simillimum.com/education/little-library. Last accessed July 2013.

Little, D. *A Comparison of the Centesimal and LM Potency Tools* http://www.simillimum.com/education/little-library. Last accessed July 2013.

Little, D. *Administering the Dose*, http://www.simillimum.com/education/little-library. Last accessed July 2013.

Little, D. *Managing the Case*, http://www.simillimum.com/education/little-library. Last accessed July 2013.

Little, D. *Preparing the Medicinal Solution*, http://www.simillimum.com/education/little-library. Last accessed July 2013.

Little, D. *The LM Potency*, http://www.simillimum.com/education/little-library. Last accessed July 2013.

Little, D. *The Medicinal Solution*, http://www.simillimum.com/education/little-library. Last accessed July 2013.

Little, D. *The 6th Organon and the Paris Casebooks*, http://www.simillimum.com/education/little-library. Last accessed July 2013.

Morgan, (1895) *Clinical Cases and Thoughts and Repetition International Hahnemann Association*, accessed in RadarOpus 2013.

Morrison, R. (1998) *Desktop Companion to Physical Pathology,* San Francisco, Hahnemann Clinic Publishing, California

Morrison, R. (1993) *Desktop Guide to Keynote & Confirmatory Symptoms,* Hahnemann Clinic Publishing, California.

Newall, P. *Rhetoric and rhetorical figures* www.galilean-library.org/int21.html. Last accessed July 2013.

Patel, P.R. (1980) *My Experiments with 50 Millesimal Scale Potencies.* Kerala: Hahnemann Homoeopathic Pharmacy, 4th ed., accessed in RadarOpus 2013.

Roberts, H.A. (1936) *The Principles and Art of Cure by Homoeopathy,* Homœopathic Publishing Co., London, accessed in RadarOpus 2013.

Rothenberg, A. (2005) *Simillimum,* accessed in RadarOpus 2013.

Russell, B. (1912) *The Problems of Philosophy,* Oxford University Press, Oxford.

Sankaran, P. (1996) *The Elements of Homoeopathy*, Homoeopathic Medical Publishers, Bombay.

Scholten, J. (2000), *Homeopathy and the Elements*, Stichting Alonnissos.

Seeley, D. *Twenty Special Forms of Rhetoric,* www.specgram.com/CXLVII.3/09.seely.rhetoric.html. Last accessed Oct 2013.

Sherr, J. (1994) Lecture. Dynamis School London.

Siegel, H. (1988) *Educating Reason: Rationality, Critical Thinking, and Education,* Routledge, New York.

Steup, M. (1996) *An Introduction to Contemporary Epistemology.* Prentice Hall.

Treuherz, F. (2010) *Genius of Homeopathy, A collection of 19th century writings on Hahnemann and homeopathy*, Saltire Books, Glasgow.

Treuherz, F. (1984) *The Origins of Kent's Homoeopathy,* Journal of the American Institute of Homoeopathy, Vol. 77 (4).

Vithoulkas, G. (1980) *The Science of Homeopathy,* Grove Press, Weidenfeld.

Watson, I. (1991) *Guide to the Methodologies of Homeopathic Prescribing*, Cutting Edge Publications, Kendell.

Weir, M. (2007) *Complementary Medicine: Ethics and Law,* Promethius Publications, Queensland.

Winston, J. (2001) *The Heritage of Homeopathic Literature,* Great Auk Publishing, Tawa.

Winston, J. (1999) *The Faces of Homeopathy,* Great Auk Publishing, Tawa.